# Liberation Plate Challenge
# COOKBOOK

## Red, Black, and Green Healing Foods

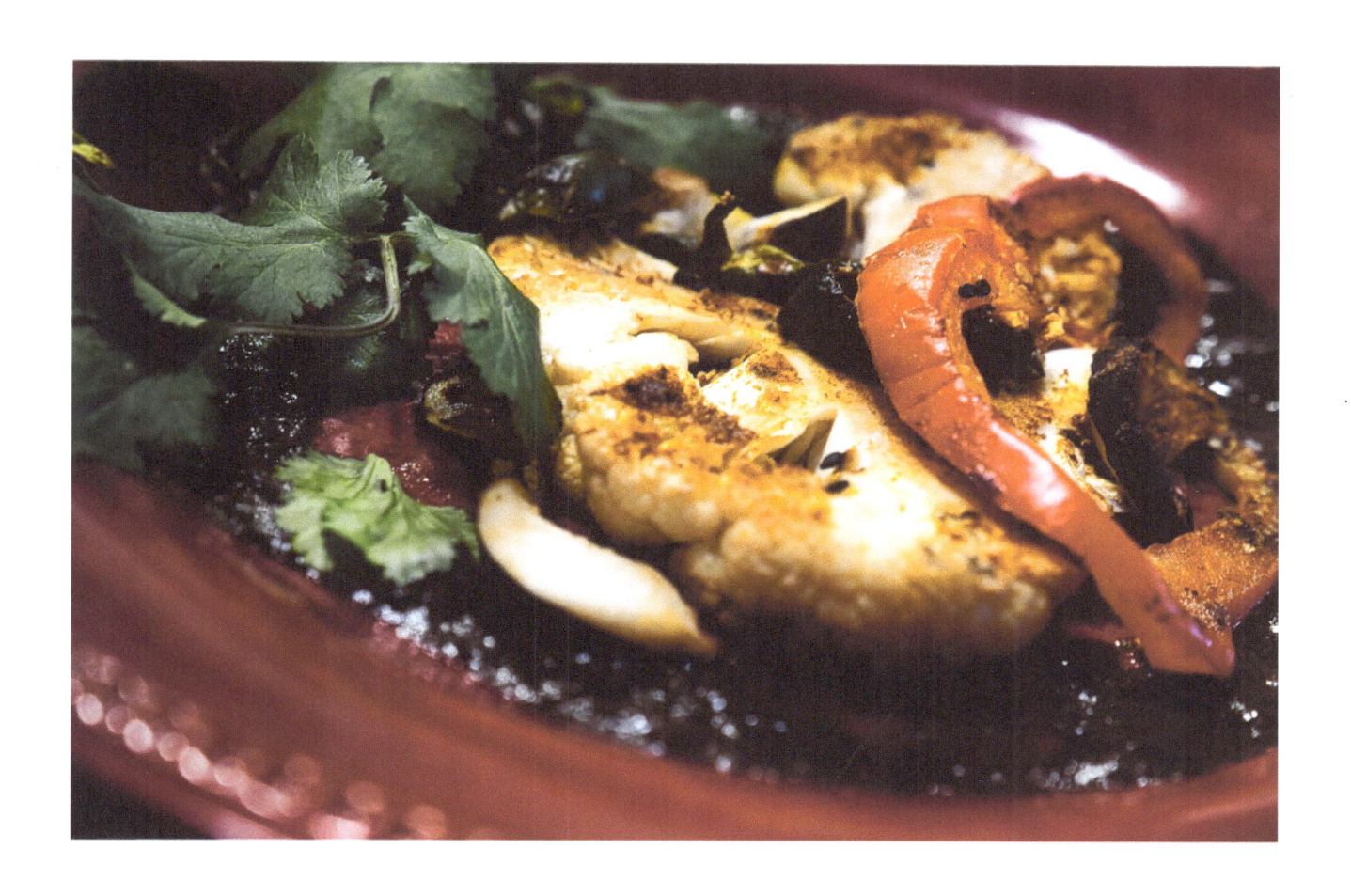

*Authors:*
**GRACE CHEPTU, AFIYA MADZIMOYO, JASMINE BARBER**

*Editor:*
**WEKESA O. MADZIMOYO**

© 2023 by AYA Educational Institute, LLC Stone Mountain, GA

Liberation Plate Challenge Cookbook
**Red**, **Black**, and **Green** Healing Foods

Copyright © 2023 by AYA Educational Institute, LLC
Grace Cheptu, Afiya Madzimoyo, Jasmine Barber, *Liberation Plate Challenge Cookbook: Red, Black and Green Healing Foods,* edited by Wekesa O. Madzimoyo

All rights reserved. No part of this publication may be reproduced, stored in a retreival system, or transmitted, in any form or by and means, electronic, mechanical, photocopying, recording or otherwise, without the prior written permission of the copyright owner.

PB ISBN: 979-8-9855646-0-0 (Hardback)
PB ISBN: 979-8-9855646-1-7 (Softback)
EB ISBN: 979-8-9855646-2-4 (E-Book)

# Dedication

We dedicate this book to AYA's Ngolo Movement, formed in March 2020 to respond to COVID-19. Hundreds worldwide embraced the Ngolo Protocols explicitly designed to enhance and sustain the body's immune response to the virus that has claimed too many. They have sacrificed, met regularly, educated themselves, and shared their discoveries and creations with family, friends, co-workers, and even strangers.

Theirs has been a path less traveled, and we salute them.

While many agencies encouraged isolation, we sought to counter the negative impact of isolation on our immune systems. Our Ngolo Protocol also encouraged us to strengthen and deepen our social connections.

Is there a better way to do that than through food? Making and sharing delicious food is one of the most social human activities, and proper nutrition is fundamental for a robust and life-saving immune response.

This Liberation cookbook is a testament to their continued work to nurture **Ngolo Zandiâkina** - our bodies' self-healing power.

The movement continues. Your purchase and your sharing ensure that it will continue to do so. Should you want to learn more or join more formally, please visit https://aya-membership-community.mn.co.


*AYA (Akan/Twi): resourcefulness, endurance, defiance (in the face of difficulty), independence.*

*Ngolo (Kikongo): strength and power*

# "Liberation Starts at Home" -- Jasmine Barber

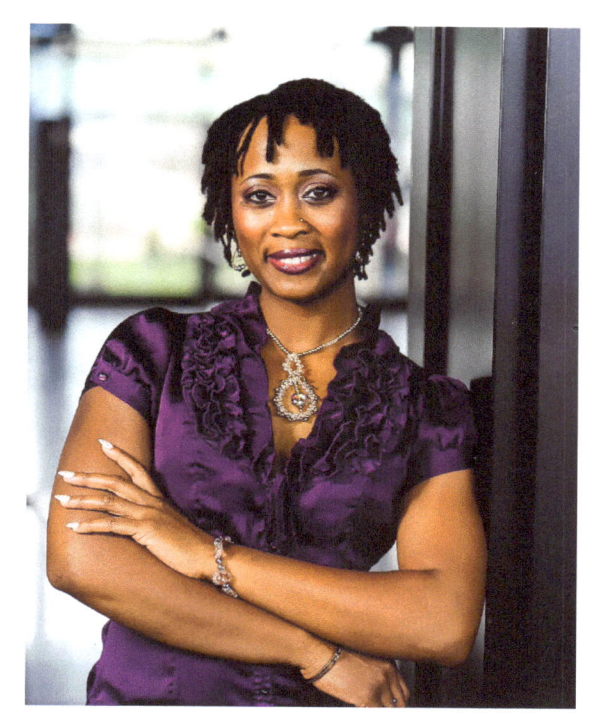

I love to cook. Preparing nourishing meals for myself and the ones I love brings my soul joy and allows me to express myself artistically. Who knew that cooking could be art? Anything you create is art. Gathering the elements, laying them out, putting them together, creating something new is the essence of artistic expression, and I thoroughly enjoy it.

In March 2020, I learned about new elements to add to my culinary creations - allomelanins or melanated foods. I learned about the extraordinary immune system boosting benefits of black foods: black rice, black garlic, black sesame seeds, blueberries, blackberries, echinacea, saw palmetto, and other allomelanins.

Before attending a series of Ngolo Town Hall meetings, I never knew about these foods. There I learned of the beauty, importance, and magnificence of our melanin in healing and protecting our beautiful bodies and what we needed to do to Feed our Blackness.

I began to add these healing foods to my cooking. Also, I began to grow healing foods in my Ngolo Garden -- garlic to make black garlic, purple basil, greens of all kinds, medicinal herbs. I wanted to be a part of my own healing and liberation from the oppression in my local food system.

I love to eat. Eating beautiful, nourishing foods that I grow in my garden and lovingly prepare is inspiring, stimulating, and liberating. As I started adding Ngolo elements to the foods I prepared for myself and my children, I thought about the liberation of Afrikans. I thought about Pan Afrikanism and the feelings of joy and power and a sense of unity with my people. I thought about our flag and the colors of our liberation.
**Red. Black. Green.**

My plates started reflecting the liberation I wanted for myself and our people.
**Red. Black. Green.**

Assorted red and green vegetable stir fry over a bed of savory black rice.
**Red. Black. Green.**

**LIBERATION PLATE CHALLENGE COOKBOOK**

Kale and spinach salad with sweet red peppers, jalapeños, and black quinoa.
**Red**. **Black**. **Green**.

Baba Wekesa Madzimoyo's leadership inspired others in our Ngolo Movement to "feed our Blackness." Mama Khem Irby, of Guilford, NC, shared a picture of what she called her Liberation Plate … a delicious red, black, and green culinary creation!

A movement was born, and in February 2021, AYA launched the Liberation Plate Challenge. We prepared and photographed **red**, **black**, and **green** dishes and shared them with others under the hashtag *#LiberationPlateChallange* on all social media!

This experience was so much fun. The energy, power, and creativity soared worldwide. We were all creating and enjoying our liberation plates despite the depression and confusion surrounding COVID19. We created our Ngolo Liberation Plates, planned our liberation gardens, and inspired one another. Through food and the spirit of liberation, we uplifted and encouraged each other.

Which is what we do as Afrikans.
**We create**. **We inspire**. **We liberate**.

Enjoy this fantastic compilation of the Spring 2021 Ngolo Liberation Plates. May you be inspired to create delicious healing meals to liberate yourself and, in doing so, liberate us all.

# "Oh, What a Challenge!" -- Grace Cheptu

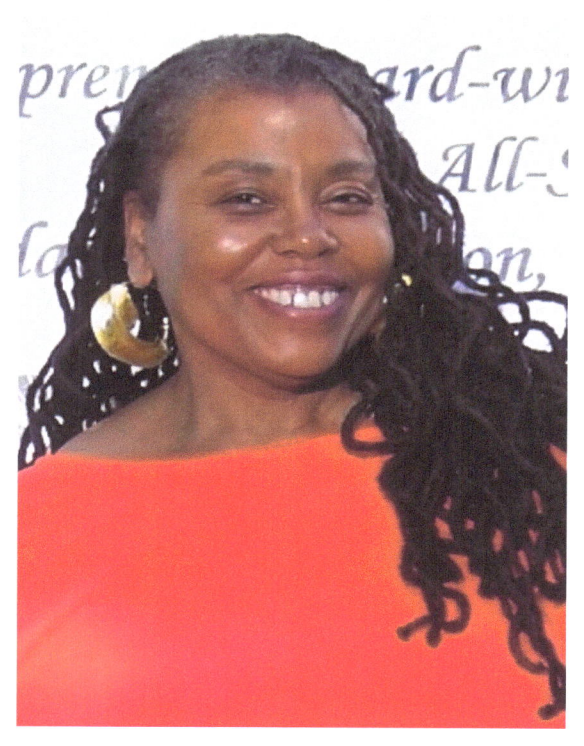

It was almost a year into the COVID-19 pandemic. I had been suffering from isolation and pandemic bloat. I felt very sad as I witnessed the loss of so many beloved national figures and loved ones close to home. And there was the continuing and most shocking loss of Black life due to police violence and the subsequent civil unrest, which evoked anger, more sadness, and grief. When I read about the #LiberationPlateChallenge, I was ready to connect with others in an intentional and life-giving way. I prepared myself to wake up my creativity and celebrate with others while building my health and a sense of personal and collective empowerment. Not to mention the celebration of my Blackness and melanin-richness down to the foods I eat…right on time!

Mama Afiya posted a video of allomelanin-rich foods she had purchased at local markets. I followed her lead and went to our local farmers market in search of as many **red**, **black,** and **green** foods as I could find. Wow, I never noticed so many choices before. I often bought brown lentils but never noticed there were also red ones and black "beluga" ones. I never noticed black rice! I'd purchased quinoa before, but never noticed there were also red and black varieties! I even saw some black flours, but uh-uh, I wasn't going to touch that…no more "bread" for these hips! I purchased my regular red beans, black beans, and organic blue corn chips, black sesame seeds, and other goodies. I stocked up on my perishables, too – beets to juice and roast; greens, greens, and more greens; eggplant, green coconuts, black plums, blackberries, kiwi fruit, and purple romaine lettuces almost too pretty to eat. Pomegranates were in season. I was having a ball!

February 1st came, my first day of the Challenge. My refrigerator was packed. Oh, my goodness! What was I thinking? Now I'll be cooking all day, every day, to cook all this stuff before it spoils! I had to get busy!

The Liberation Challenge was a LOT of fun as I honored familiar foods from my Gullah ancestral roots and experimented with new foods and flavor combinations. At first, it was more about making pretty **red**, **black**, and **green** plates; then I began to shift my focus toward the healing properties and combination of my foods and spices. I rehabilitated my herb garden that had gone kaput. I became more aware of the fiber content from the abundance of my veggies, fruits, nuts, and seeds.

The Challenge said nothing about vegetarianism or the consumption of animal proteins … simply **red**, **black**, and **green**. As I became focused on experimenting with new foods and using up all my fresh veggies and fruit, I hadn't noticed that I had practically stopped eating animal protein, except occasional seafood. I discovered that I could enjoy completely satisfying meals day after day without meat. I also found that making my plates "pretty" made me appreciate my meals much more. Seeing the beauty of the meals and foods others posted in the Challenge filled me with happiness. I could feel the love on their plates and in their stories.

After just one week of the Challenge, I began to feel better. I had more energy as my body began to purge and cleanse. My skin was glowing by the end of the month, and my eyes cleared. What a way to celebrate and begin a new, more nutrition-conscious lifestyle and have fun while doing it! Thanks to the team that came up with such a clever idea! And then, it hit me…we need to make a cookbook!

# "A Game Changer" -- Afiya Madzimoyo

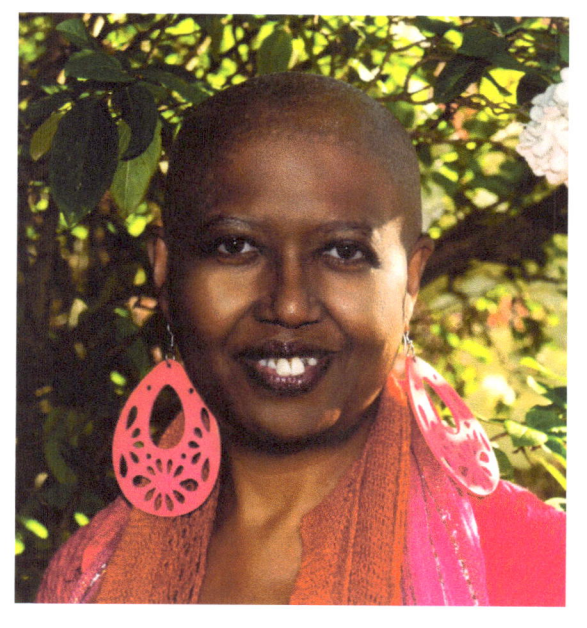

Just the idea of our #LiberationPlateChallenge was empowering. Mama Khem first mentioned flag plates, and I thought Italian red, green, and white. I remember thinking, "Let's use our (Garvey) flag," and in no time, we were praising the **red**, **black**, and **green** on our plates.

I decided the easiest way to embrace this Challenge was to go out and purchase all the **red**, **black**, and **green** foods I could find at our local farmer's market. At the Asian market, I found black sesame seeds, black noodles, and dried black neem leaves.

So inspired by Mama Qoqo's weekly green drink embellished with a red ribbon, I purchased **red**, **black**, and **green** plates and bowls. Her green drink inspired my *Juiced up for Toning* Challenge entry. *Mama Cheptu's Morning Berry Tonic* took me over the top. Bitten by the #LiberationPlateChallenge bug, I began posting nearly every day of the Challenge. Somehow I managed to post even when I was traveling.

Seeing all the healthy and beautifully plated entries come in every day excited my soul. It was like a call and response show. I would see a post and just become enlivened and inspired to produce something healthy and dazzling. Mama Jasmine posted her beautiful "Mayan Superfood Oatmeal," and memories of the warmth and love of my mom's oatmeal flooded in. That deluge resulted in one of my favorite entries: *Not My Mama's Oatmeal* made with chia seeds soaked overnight.

Each dish energized me to produce **red**, **black**, and **green** foods with as many allomellanins as possible. So now, when I shop, I'm looking for black sesame seeds, black garlic, black rice, black tomatoes, blackberries, and black activated charcoal - a great accomplishment in and of itself.

I have always loved to cook my Grandma Muh's collard greens - just like she did with a pinch of this and a touch of that. It was a challenge and a delight to convert her pinches and touches into a more easily quantifiable recipe. I succeeded except when converting a "mess" of collards into cups or pounds. You are on your own there. A "mess" is still a mess, and you'll feel your way through it.

LIBERATION PLATE CHALLENGE COOKBOOK

Throughout all my years of cooking, I have never been that particular about "plating." I'm very fast at prepping and preparing/cooking food in my mama's tradition. In fact, I never intend to be in the kitchen for more than an hour or so. Seeing the beautiful **RBG** plates, I upped my game. Wekesa, my husband, says I'm a changed woman when it comes to how I present food now, and he ain't nev'a lied.

Mama Cheptu says it became a competition, and it did in an excellent, healthy way. In AYA's **7 Steps to Recovery, it's called** self-to-other comparison, and we are encouraged to compare our results to those of others for information and inspiration. "How did they do that!?" "That is beautiful," and through my eyes, I could taste the plate.

I ate better throughout the #LiberationPlateChallenge. Primarily because of many of the challenges of COVID, I connected with my NGOLO family in a remarkable way that fed me on all levels: physically, mentally, emotionally, and spiritually. This call and response to produce healthy **red**, **black** and **green** plates netted us over 100 entries and remarkable benefits that will support us individually and collectively as a people for years and years to come.

# Table of Contents

*Dedication* ............................................................................................................. 5

*"Liberation Starts at Home" -- Jasmine Barber* ............................................... 7

*"Oh, What a Challenge!" -- Grace Cheptu* ...................................................... 9

*"A Game Changer" -- Afiya Madzimoyo* ........................................................ 11

## SECTION I: LIBERATION TONICS, SMOOTHIES AND PORRIDGES ................. 16

    Juiced Up for Toning, Cleansing and Building ............................................ 18

    Morning Berry Tonic ...................................................................................... 19

    Mornin' Immune Boosting Tea ...................................................................... 20

    Sun-Infused Strawberry/Lavender Water .................................................... 21

    Quick and Green Apple Cider ........................................................................ 22

    Beet Juice, Banana and Fruit Smoothie Bowl ............................................. 23

    Green Coconut Water Smoothie and Fruit .................................................. 24

    Green Smoothie Bowl .................................................................................... 25

    Mayan Superfood Oatmeal ............................................................................ 26

    Not My Mama's Oatmeal ............................................................................... 28

    Raw Mamey Sapote Pie ................................................................................. 29

## SECTION II: LIBERATION SALADS, SOUPS AND SNACKS .............................. 31

    My Favorite Salad .......................................................................................... 32

    Red Quinoa Avocado Salad ........................................................................... 34

    Arugula Spinach Salad with Vinaigrette ...................................................... 36

    Lacinato Kale and Swiss Chard Salad ......................................................... 37

    Mama Makes Ends Avocado Salad .............................................................. 39

    Liberation Kale Salad .................................................................................... 40

    Big Raw Lunch Salad with Butterhead Lettuce and Alfalfa Sprouts ......... 42

    Black Goddess Watermelon Avocado Salad ............................................... 43

    Spring Strawberry Salad ............................................................................... 44

Salad Fruity Nutty Seedy ........................................................................................... 46

Pomegranate Vinaigrette .......................................................................................... 47

RBG Fruit Plate ......................................................................................................... 48

Red Lentil Soup with Roasted Tomatoes and Red Peppers ................................... 49

Black Bean Soup with Tomatoes and Fresh Spinach ............................................. 51

Snack Time! .............................................................................................................. 53

Roasted Veggie Snack ............................................................................................. 54

Fruit-Nut-Seed Snack ............................................................................................... 56

## SECTION III: ALLOMELANINS ON DECK ........................................................... 57

Black Rice/Forbidden Rice ....................................................................................... 58

Black Garlic ............................................................................................................... 60

Black Sesame Seeds ............................................................................................... 62

Black Seed Oil/Kalonji .............................................................................................. 64

Purple Sweet Potato ................................................................................................. 66

Black Tomatoes ........................................................................................................ 68

Saw Palmetto ............................................................................................................ 70

Mulberries ................................................................................................................. 72

Blueberries ................................................................................................................ 74

Blackberries .............................................................................................................. 76

Activated Charcoal ................................................................................................... 77

## SECTION IV: LIBERATION ENTREES, MAIN COURSES AND MEALS ............. 79

Black-Eye Peas ........................................................................................................ 80

Blueprint for Black Love Dinner ............................................................................... 83

Black Rice with Roasted Vegetables ....................................................................... 85

Grandma Muh's Southern Smothered Collard Greens ........................................... 87

Roasted Cauliflower Steak with Poblano Peppers .................................................. 89

Artichoke Pizza with Love ........................................................................................ 91

Sassy Vegan Pizza .................................................................................................. 92

Pan-Seared Salmon with Black Bean Pasta and Salad ......................................... 93

Homemade Alternative for Store-bought Vegan Cream Cheese ............................... 95

Liberation Tian: Eggplant, Tomato, Zucchini .............................................................. 96

Steamed Mussels in Garlic and White Wine Sauce ..................................................... 98

Black Pad Thai Noodles and Stir Fried Vegetables....................................................... 100

Grilled Portobello Mushrooms with Avocado Chimichurri .......................................... 102

Vegan Stir Fry ................................................................................................................ 104

Hopi's Yummy Plate ...................................................................................................... 106

Kimchi Black Fried Rice with Black Beans and Organic Pea Leaves ........................... 108

"Barbecued" Tofu with Grilled Asparagus and Black Rice ........................................... 110

**BACK COVER**................................................................................................................ 112

# Section I:
# Liberation Tonics, Smoothies, and Porridges

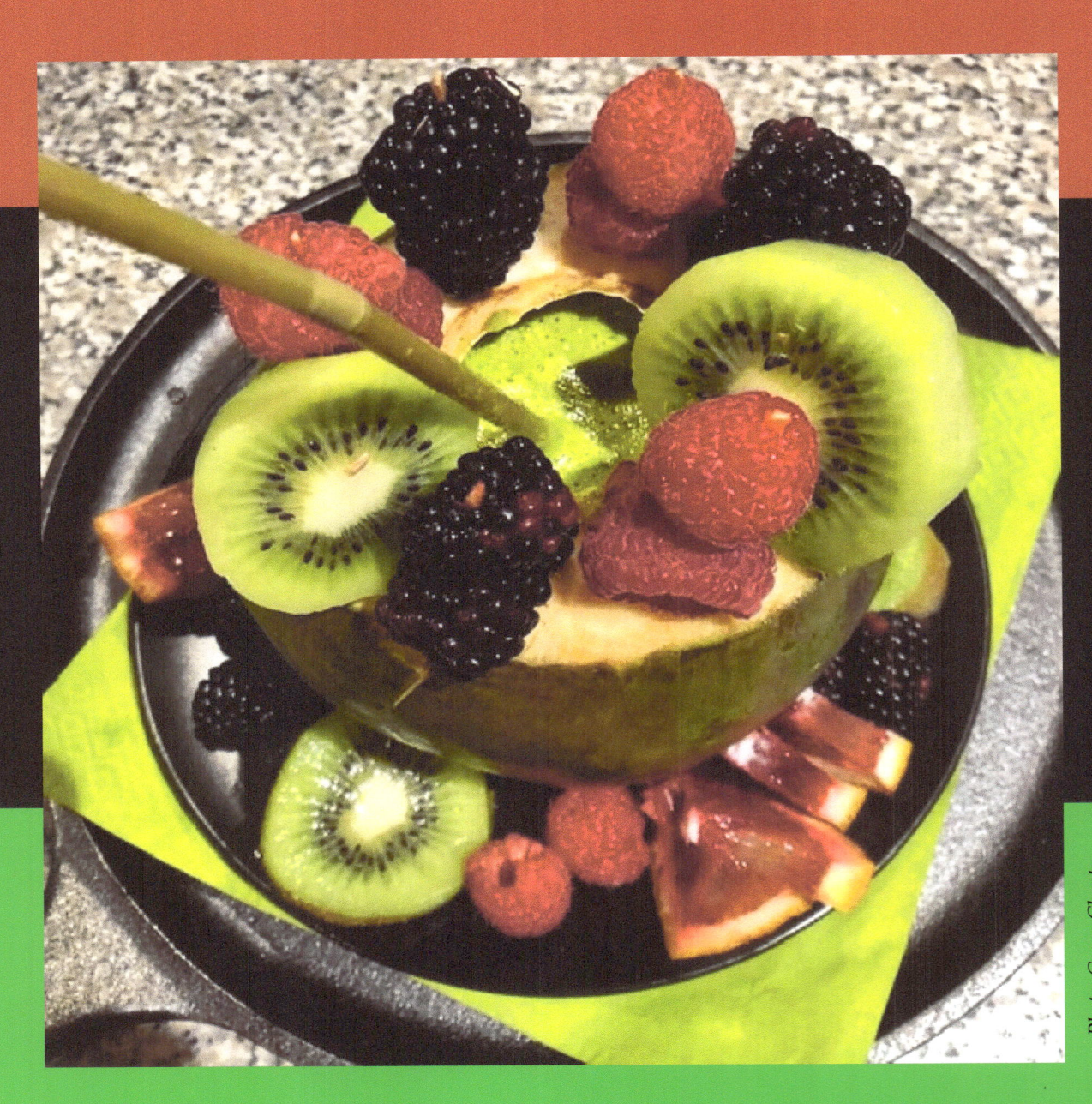

*Photo: Grace Cheptu*

# Weekly Green Drink

## Mama Qoqo

I celebrate the **Red**, the **Black**, and the **Green** as I lean into and accept the opportunity, challenge, and transformation in healing myself through the foods I eat.

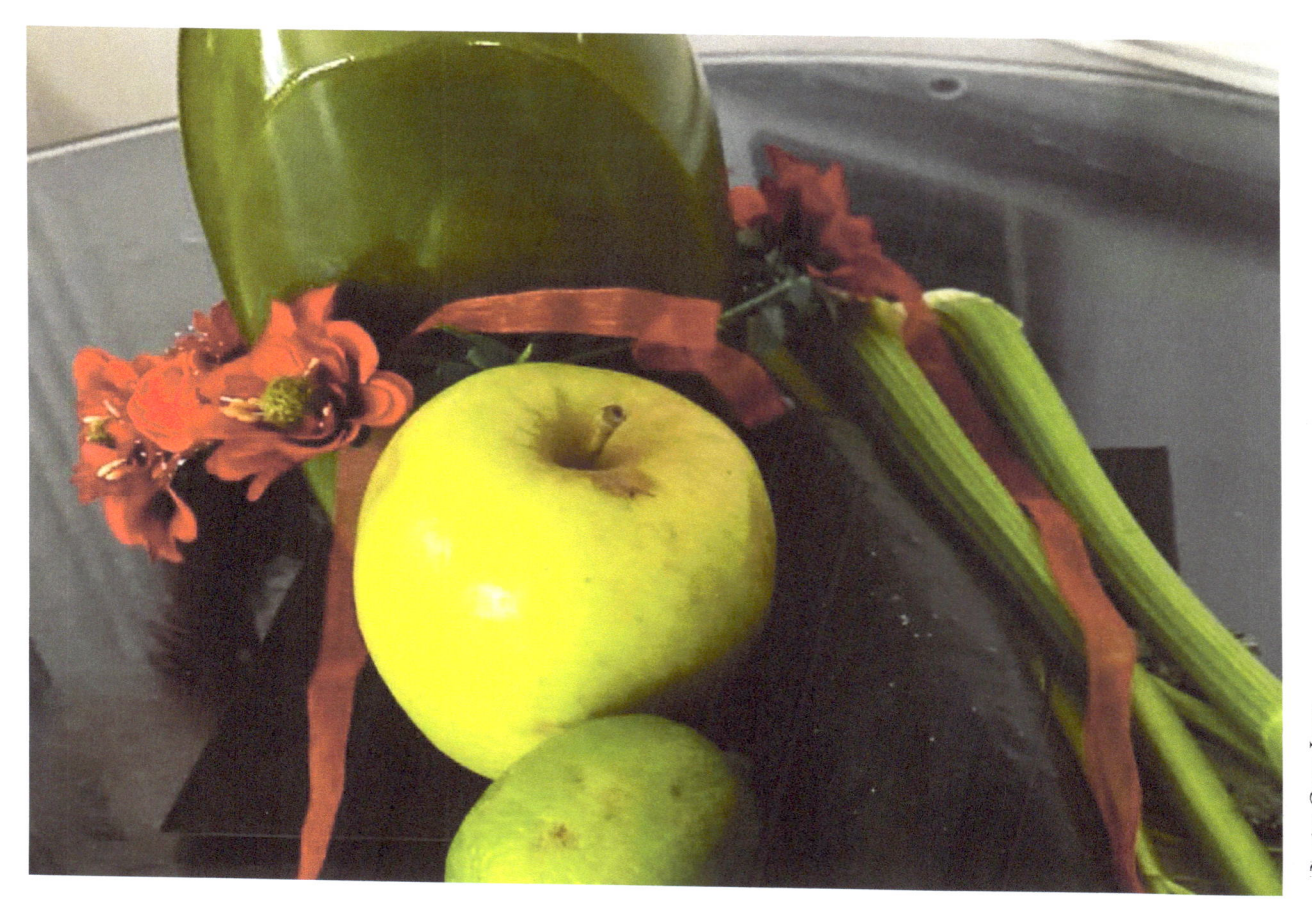

Celery, green apple, cucumber, lime. I also added ginger.

LIBERATION PLATE CHALLEN

# Juiced Up for Toning, Cleansing and Building

## Mama Afiya

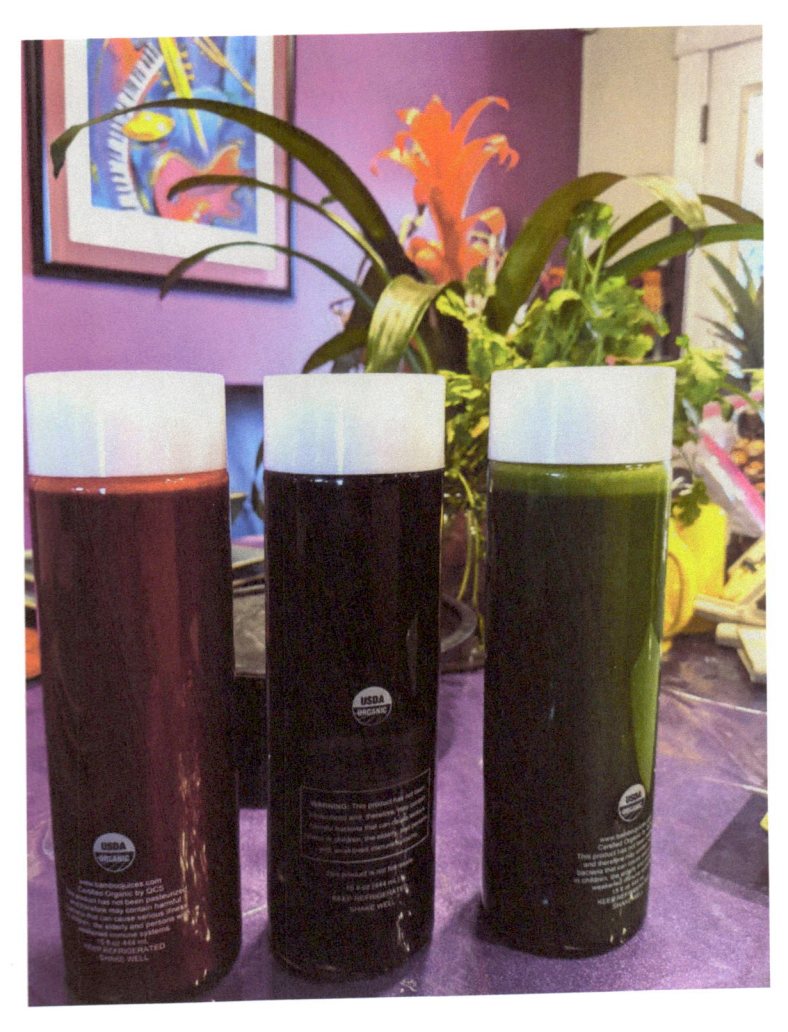

*Photo: Afiya Madzimoyo*

**RED** beets, pomegranates, red apple, turmeric, and ginger
**BLACK** ¼ teaspoon activated charcoal in water
**GREEN** kale, celery, collards, green apple

# Morning Berry Tonic

## Mama Cheptu

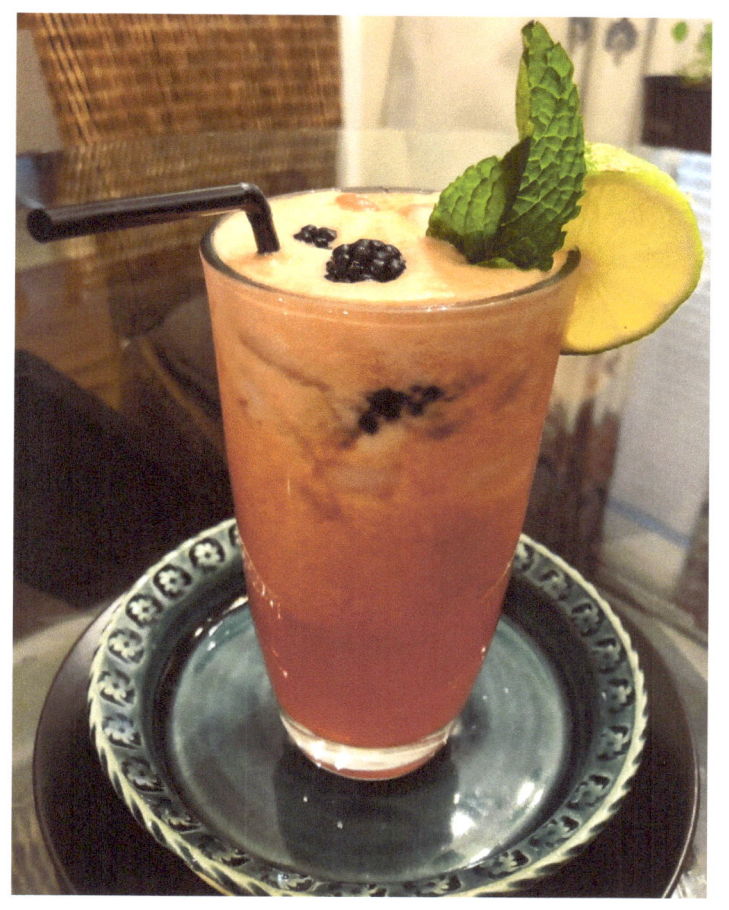

*Photo: Grace Cheptu*

**RED** raspberries and strawberries
**BLACK** peppercorns and whole blackberries
**GREEN** apple freshly juiced, spearmint leaf

Other ingredients: ginger, lemon, optional organic maple syrup. Also good with juiced raw pineapple, though not included here.

# Mornin' Immune Boosting Tea

## Mama Qoqo

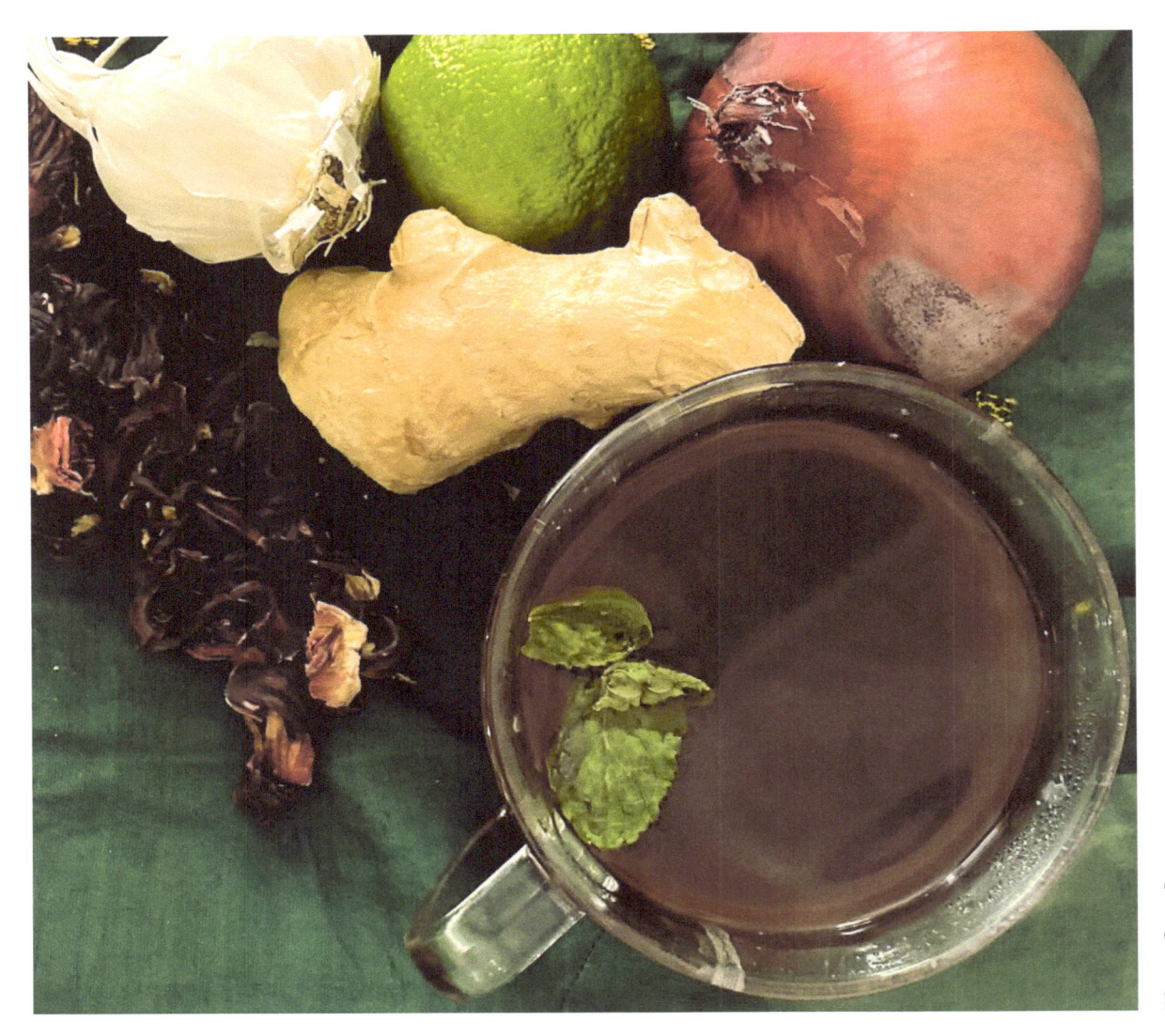

Dried hibiscus flowers, red onion, lime, ginger, garlic, mint leaf

# Sun-Infused Strawberry/Lavender Water

## Mama Afiya

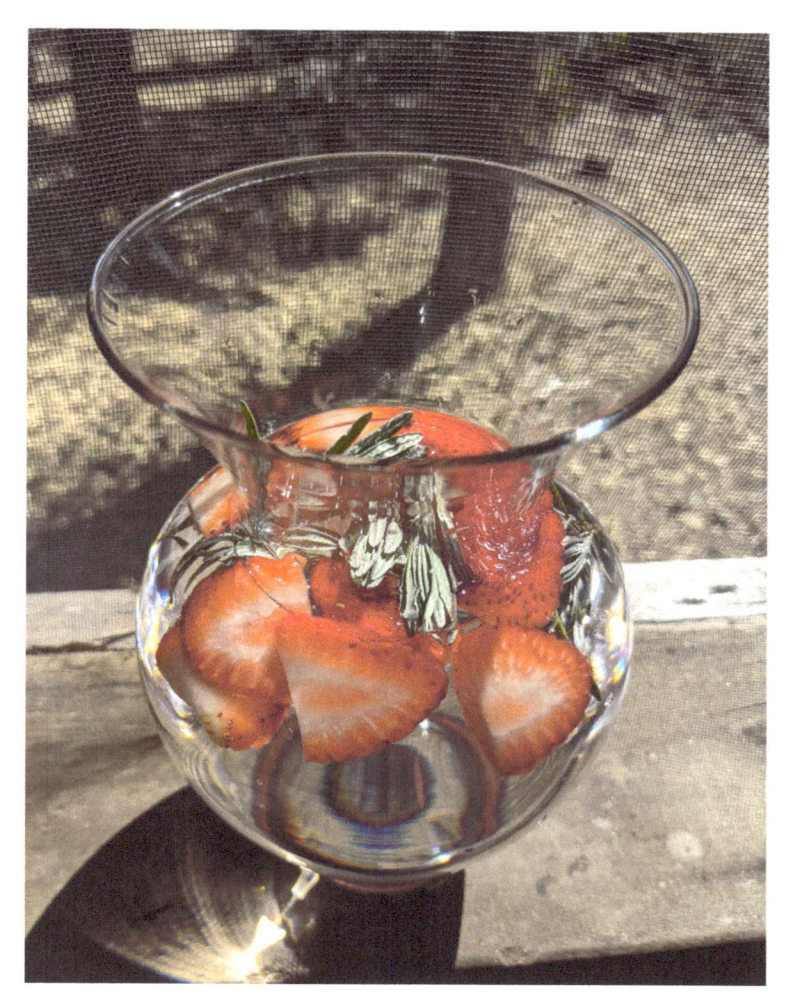

*Photo: Afiya Madzimoyo*

Your water of choice infused with strawberries, lavender, and sunshine!

# Quick and Green Apple Cider

## Mama Afiya

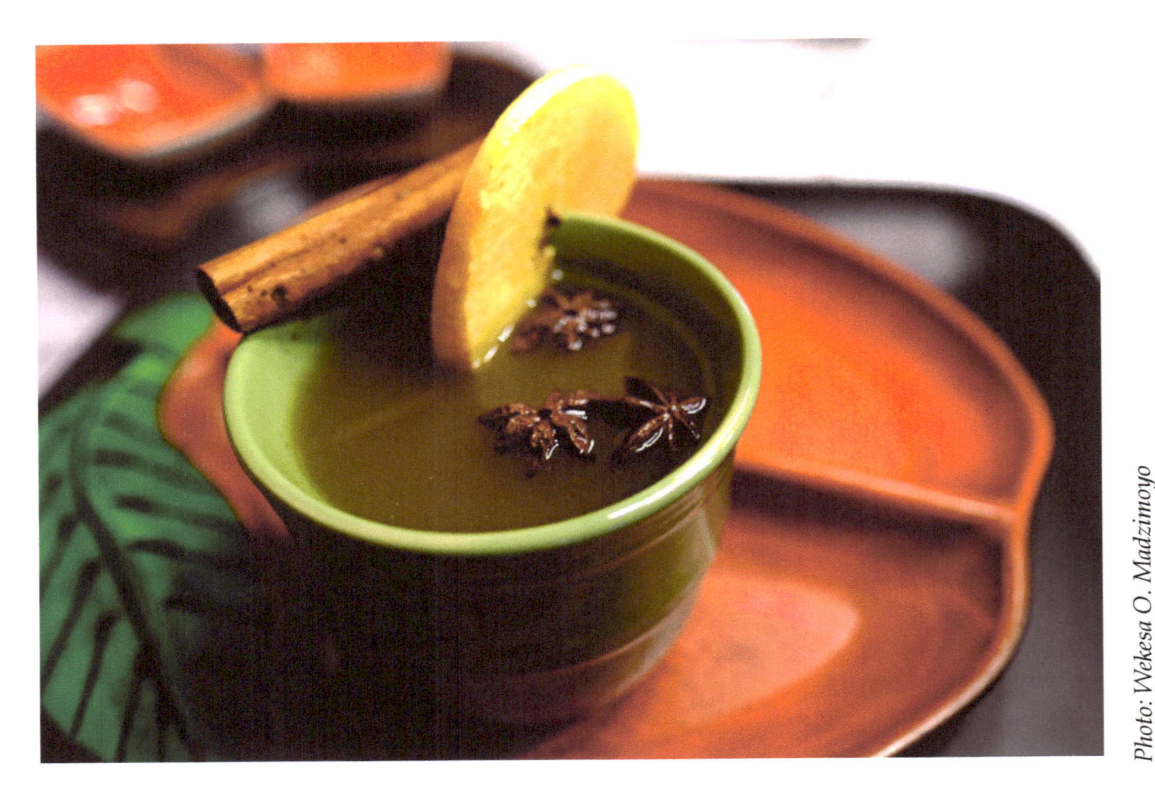

*Photo: Wekesa O. Madzimoyo*

*When it's cold outside, this joint delivers. It's sweet and nice with lots of spice, and oh, did I mention the warmth it brings down "to the bones."*

## Ingredients

- 4 large fuji apples or sweet apples of your choice juiced
- 6-8 Leaves of Life, juiced
- Pinch of cinnamon
- Few whole cloves
- Freshly ground nutmeg ( I use my grater)
- A few stars of anise

## Directions

Let all ingredients simmer on low heat for at least 20-30 minutes, so the spices have time to marry. Strain to take out some of the froth and pieces of spices. Pour into your favorite mug and garnish with an apple slice, a few stars of anise, and a cinnamon stick.

# Beet Juice, Banana, and Fruit Smoothie Bowl

## Mama Afiya

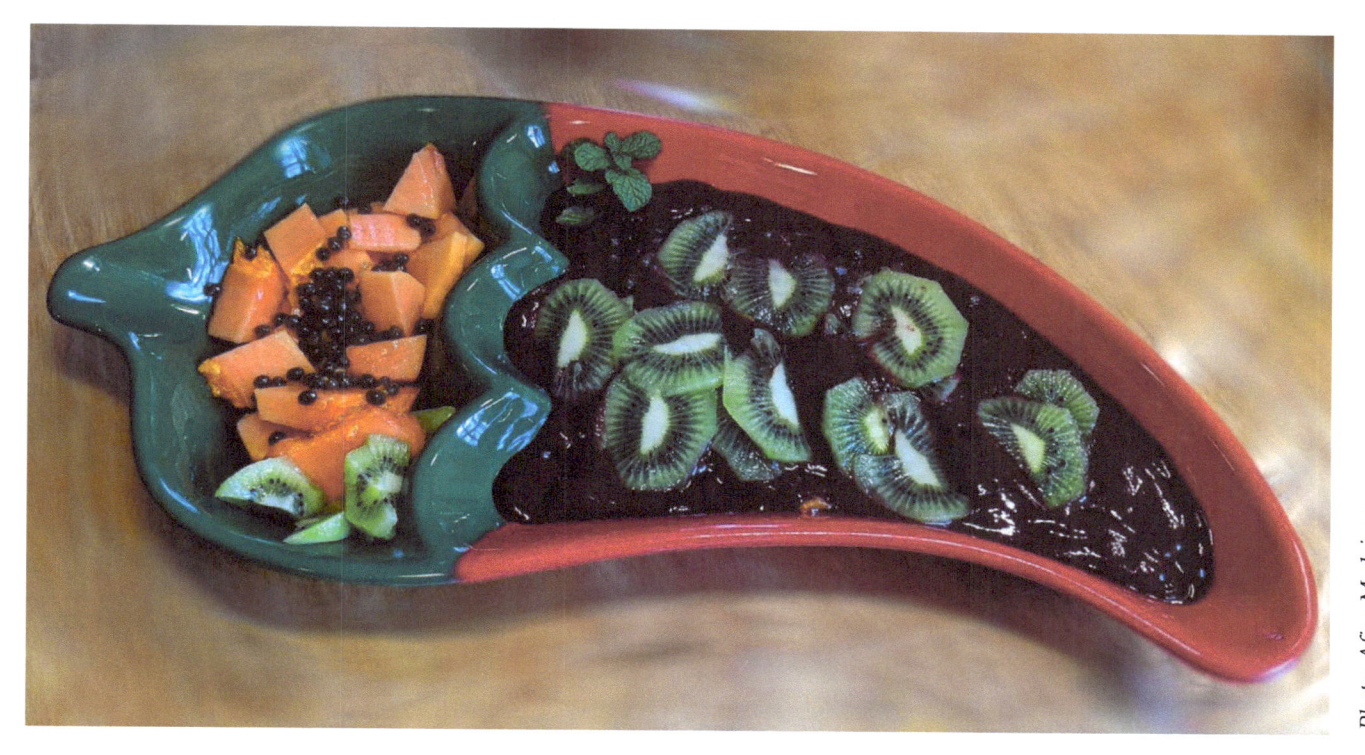

*Photo: Afiya Madzimoyo*

Smoothie made of beet juice, bananas, and blueberries. Topped with papaya, kiwifruit, and can you see the black papaya seeds? They're good for worms, parasites, and viruses.

# Green Coconut Water Smoothie and Fruit

## Mama Cheptu

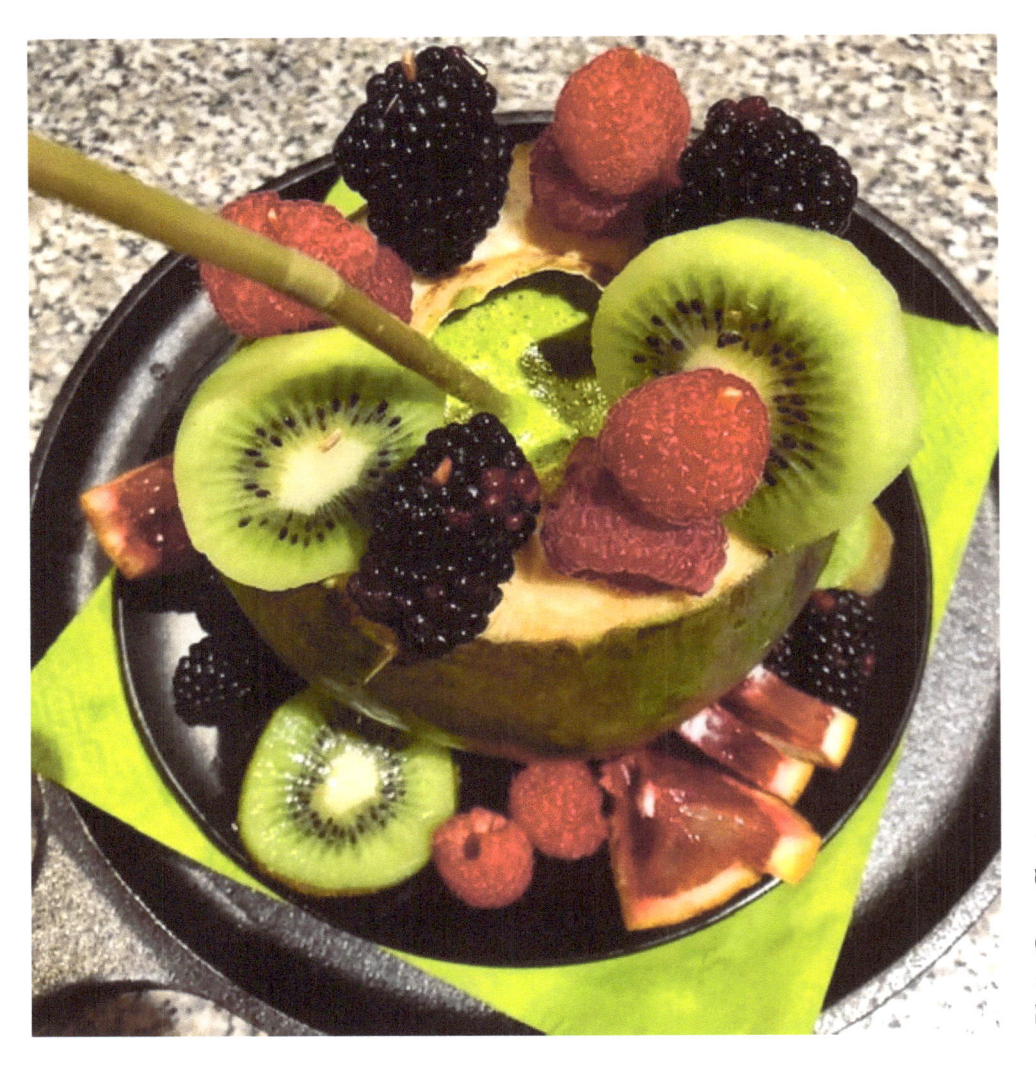

*Photo: Grace Cheptu*

Green smoothie: fresh coconut water, spinach or other greens, frozen banana, avocado (optional), lemon, ginger, and a pinch of organic maple syrup. Served in a green coconut shell and garnished with blackberries, blood orange, raspberries, kiwifruit.

# Green Smoothie Bowl

## Mama Afiya

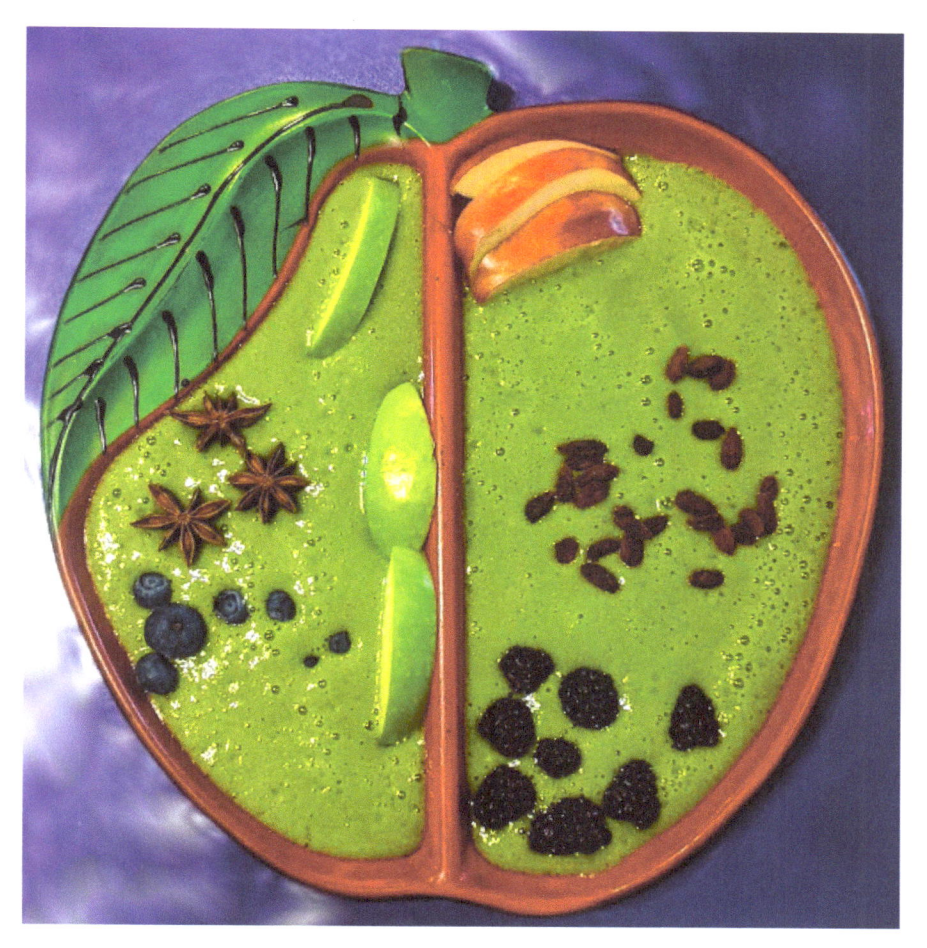

*Photo: Afiya Madzimoyo*

Greens from the garden: kale, mustard, collard, swiss chard, or any other green leafy veggie including parsley and cilantro. Water; for sweetener: one green apple or frozen banana to make it sweeter. To make it more nutritious and creamy: hemp seeds and sea moss. Top with blackberries, blueberries, goji berries, star anise, green and red apple slices.

# *Mayan Superfood Oatmeal*

## Mama Jasmine

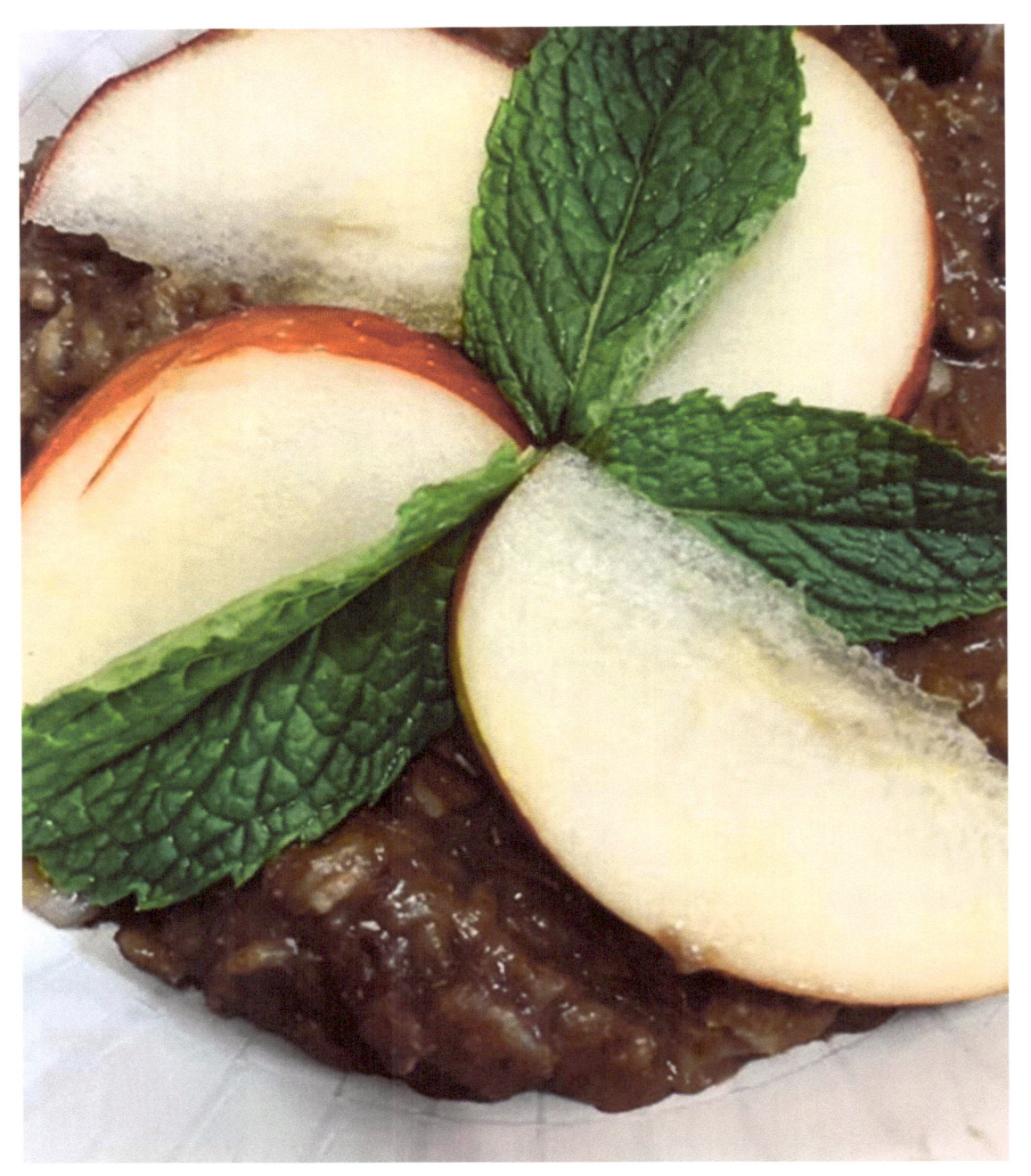

*Photo: Jasmine Barber*

## Ingredients:

- Mayan SuperFood Oatmeal by Earnest Eats (https://www.earnesteats.com) or create your own oatmeal blend with whole rolled oats, quinoa, amaranth, pepitas, sunflower seeds, chopped cashews, chopped almonds, raw flax seeds, unsweetened cocoa, Korintje cinnamon
- Organic chocolate hemp milk or plant-based milk of your choice
- 1 Honey Crisp apple
- Fresh organic mint

## Directions:

Simmer dry ingredients in chocolate hemp milk for 15-20 minutes or until soft and creamy. Stir frequently and add more hemp milk as needed to keep the creamy consistency.

Thinly slice Honey Crisp apples and place them on top along with fresh organic mint or any other topping of your choice.

# Not My Mama's Oatmeal

## Mama Afiya

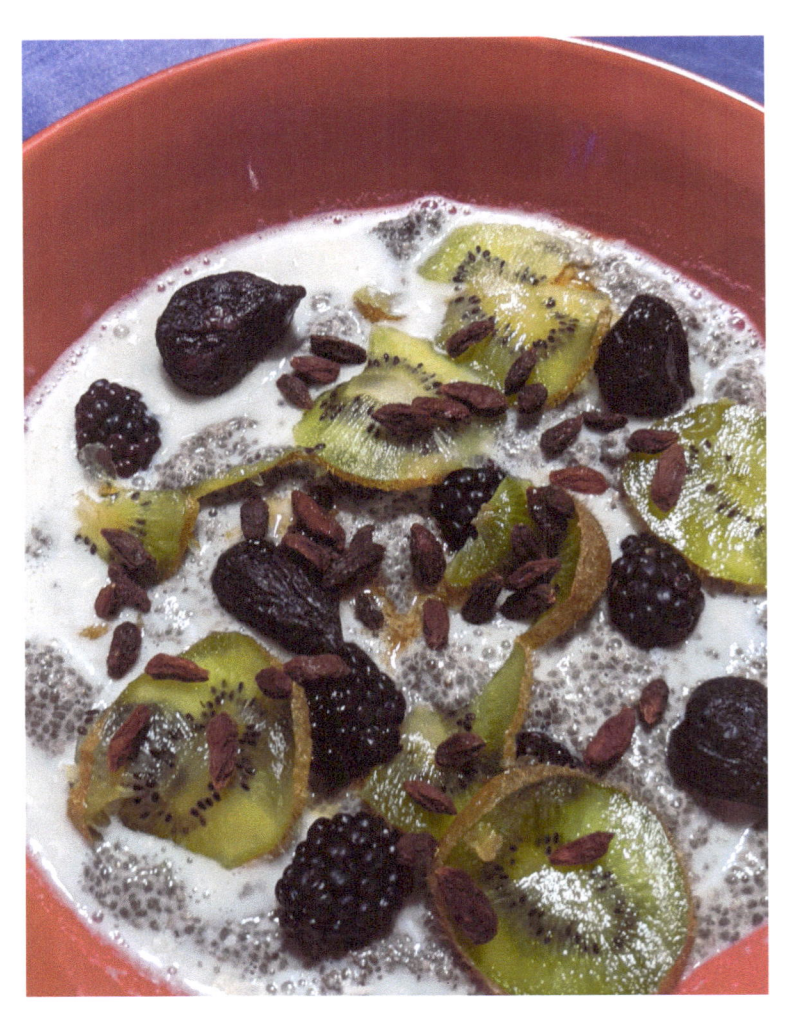

*Photo: Afiya Madzimoyo*

Soak black chia seeds overnight in almond, oat, or your favorite plant-based milk on the counter to have it at room temperature. In the morning, add kiwifruit, blackberries, black mission figs, goji berries, ground cinnamon, cloves, cardamom, and a dash of vanilla extract.

# Raw Mamey Sapote Pie

## Mama Afiya

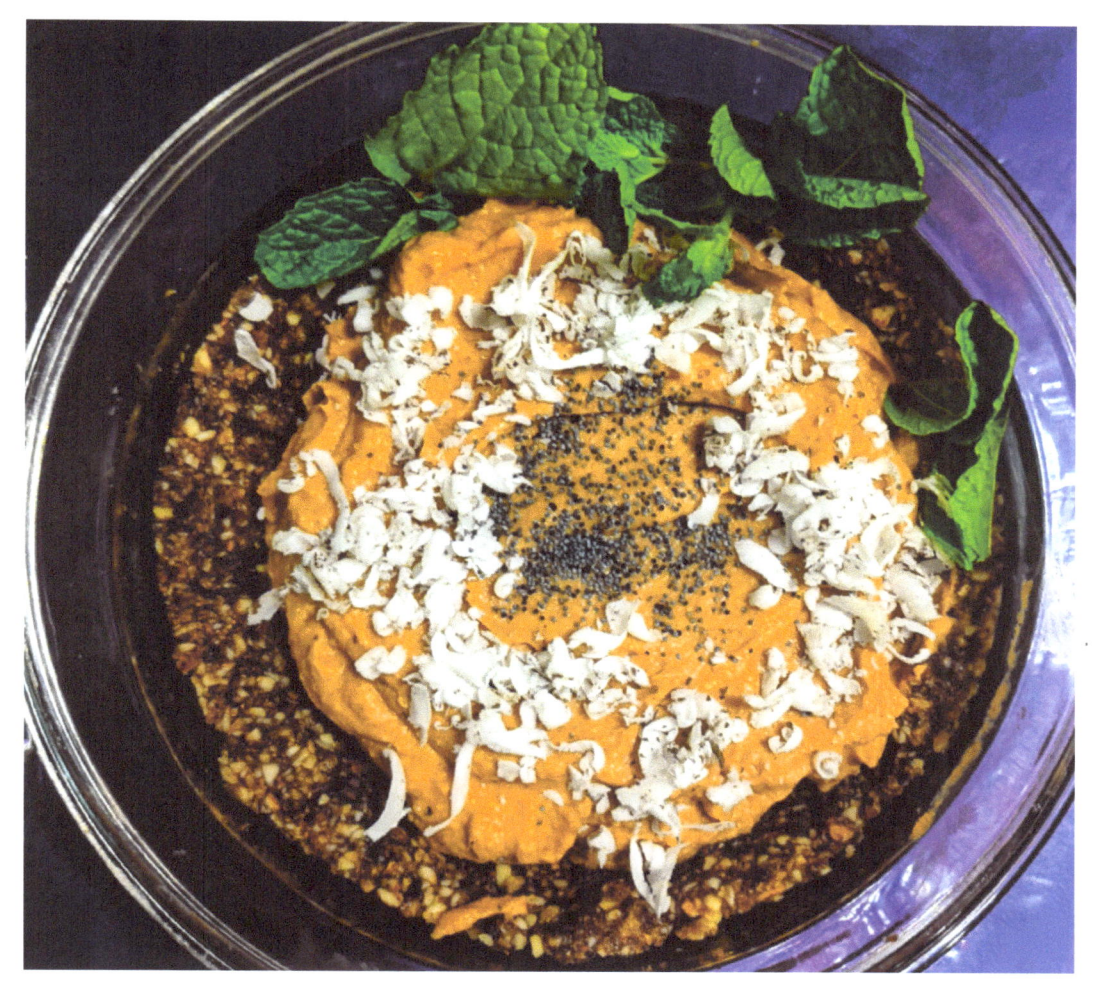

*Photo: Afiya Madzimoyo*

*Cravin' sweet potato pie, and you're staying out of the "white girls" processed sugar and dairy? Meet "mamey," who, in her raw form, tastes and feels like sweet potato custard. Enjoy!*

## Ingredients for crust:

- 1 cup pitted dates
- 1 cup almonds
- 1 teaspoon orange zest
- 2-4 tablespoons of water or brewed chai tea

## Ingredients for filling:

- 1 large, very ripe mamey sapote
- 1 tablespoon fresh ginger, minced
- 2 cups coconut cream or coconut manna
- 1½ teaspoons cinnamon
- ¼ teaspoon nutmeg
- ¼ teaspoon cloves
- ⅛ teaspoon salt
- unsweetened shredded coconut
- black poppy seeds
- spearmint leaves

## Directions:

Put all of the crust ingredients, except the water/tea, in a food processor and pulse several times. The mixture should be pretty crumbly. Scrape down the sides and add the liquid one tablespoon at a time, pulsing in between, until the consistency is semi-moist and malleable.

Plop your crust into a pie pan, and using a fork or spatula, spread it evenly over the surface and up the sides. Try to keep the thickness as even as possible.

Put all of the filling ingredients into a food processor and mix thoroughly for the filling.

Get fancy at the end and garnish with unsweetened shredded coconut, poppy seeds, and spearmint leaves.

# Section II:

## Liberation Salads, Soups, and Snacks

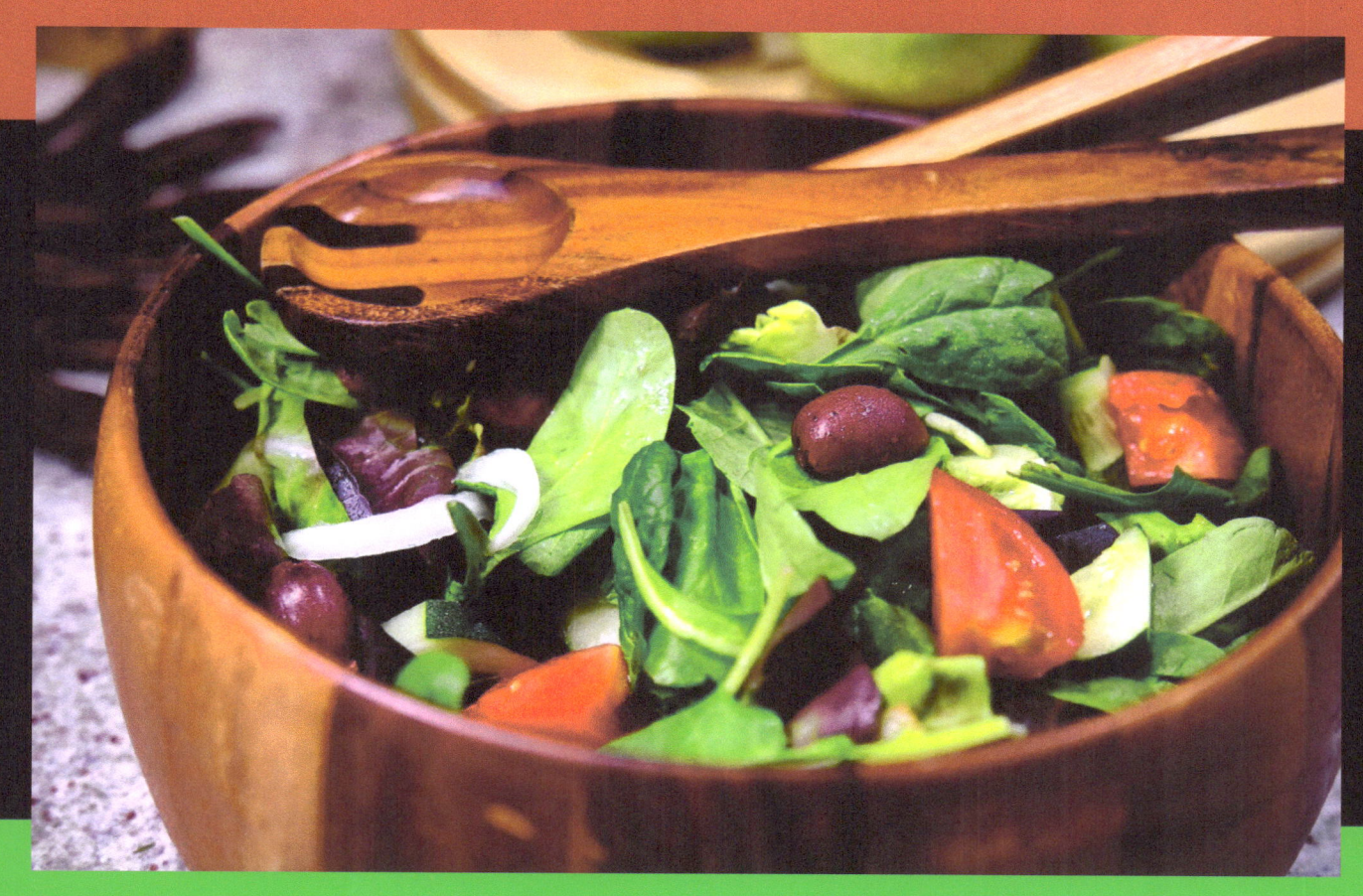

*Photo: Wekesa O. Madzimoyo*

# *My Favorite Salad*

## Mama Khem

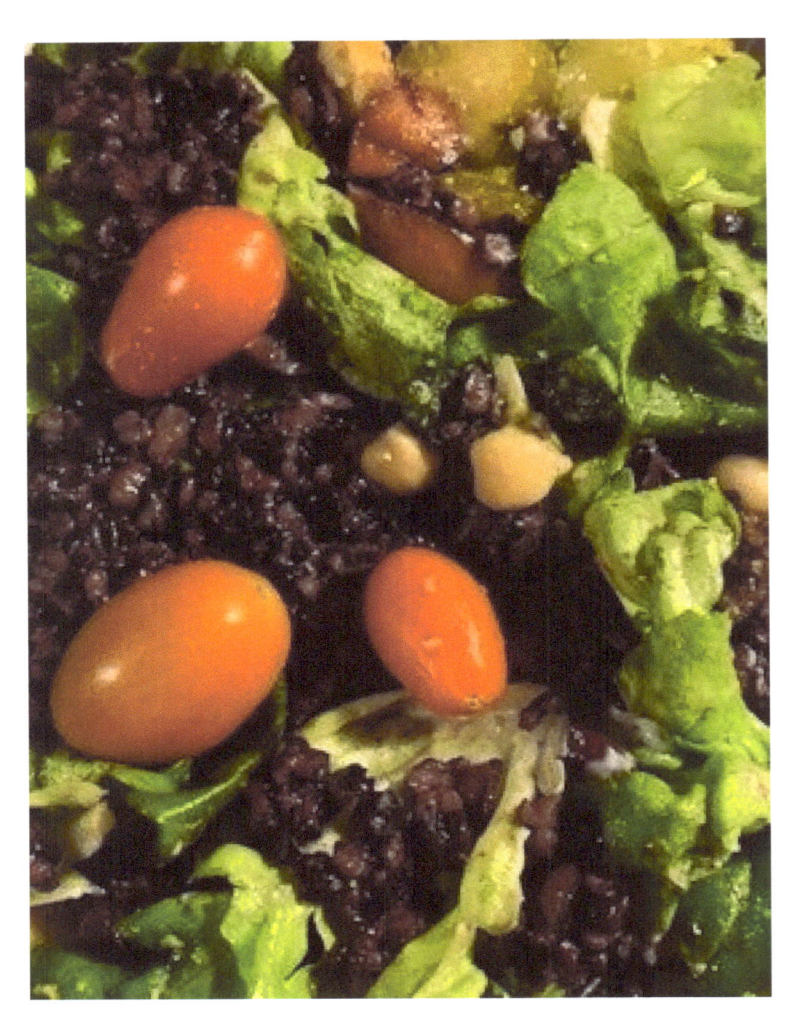

*Photo: Khem Irby*

*This is my Liberation Salad. The main ingredients must be **red**, **black**, and **green**. I cooked the black rice with black seed oil, red peppers, and garlic with a black pepper dash. The greens are called oakleaf lettuce. There are chickpeas and sweet pickles. I like my salad warm.*

# Hubby Melvin Irby's Dressing

## Ingredients:

- ¼ cup soy sauce
- ¼ cup rice wine vinegar
- 2 tablespoons minced ginger
- 2 tablespoons brown sugar
- ¾ tablespoons sesame oil
- Pinch of pepper flakes
- 2 cloves minced garlic
- ⅔ cup olive oil

## Directions:

Place all items into a blender and blend until smooth.

# Red Quinoa Avocado Salad

## Mama Cheptu

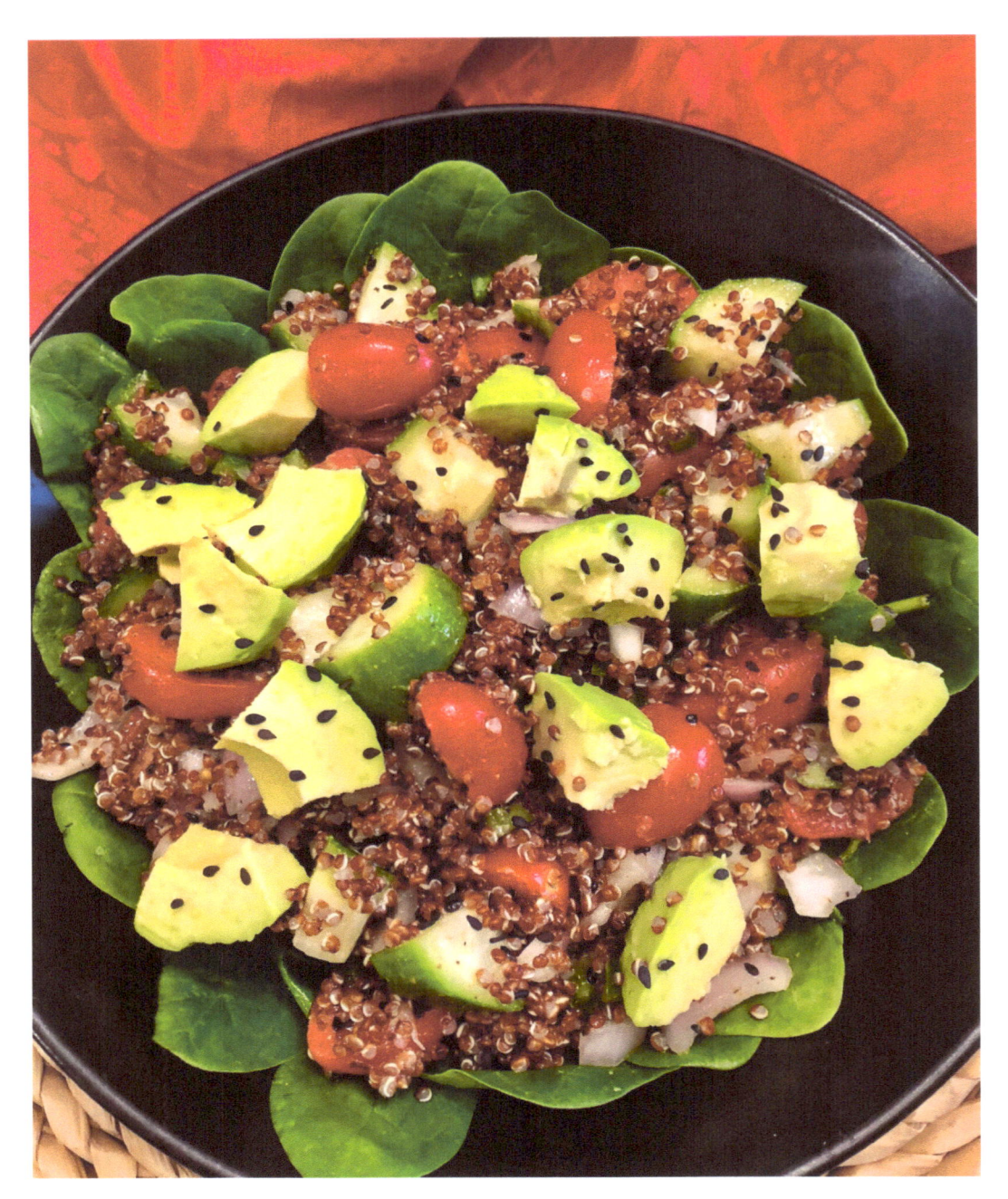

*Photo: Grace Cheptu*

## Ingredients:

- ⅓ cup organic red quinoa
- ⅔ cup water
- 1 cup cherry tomatoes, sliced in half
- ½ cup diced cucumber
- ¼ cup diced red onion
- ½ medium jalapeno pepper, finely chopped
- 3 tablespoons lime juice
- 1 tablespoon extra virgin olive oil
- ½ teaspoon ground cumin
- 2 cups baby spinach
- 1 avocado
- Salt/pepper to taste
- Black cumin or black sesame seeds

## Directions:

Rinse and drain quinoa thoroughly to remove the bitter coating.

Bring quinoa and water to a boil over high heat. Reduce heat to medium-low; cover and simmer until the quinoa is tender. After simmering for about 15 - 20 minutes, the quinoa will absorb the water. Fluff with a fork. Spread the quinoa into a bowl and refrigerate until cold (about 30 minutes).

Once the quinoa has chilled, gently stir in the tomatoes, cucumber, jalapeno pepper, and onion. Gently stir in lime juice, olive oil, cumin, salt, and pepper. Taste and adjust seasonings. Divide the spinach leaves onto salad plates, and top with the quinoa salad. Garnish with the avocado chunks or slices and lightly sprinkle with black cumin or black sesame seeds.

# Arugula Spinach Salad with Vinaigrette

## Baba Baoku

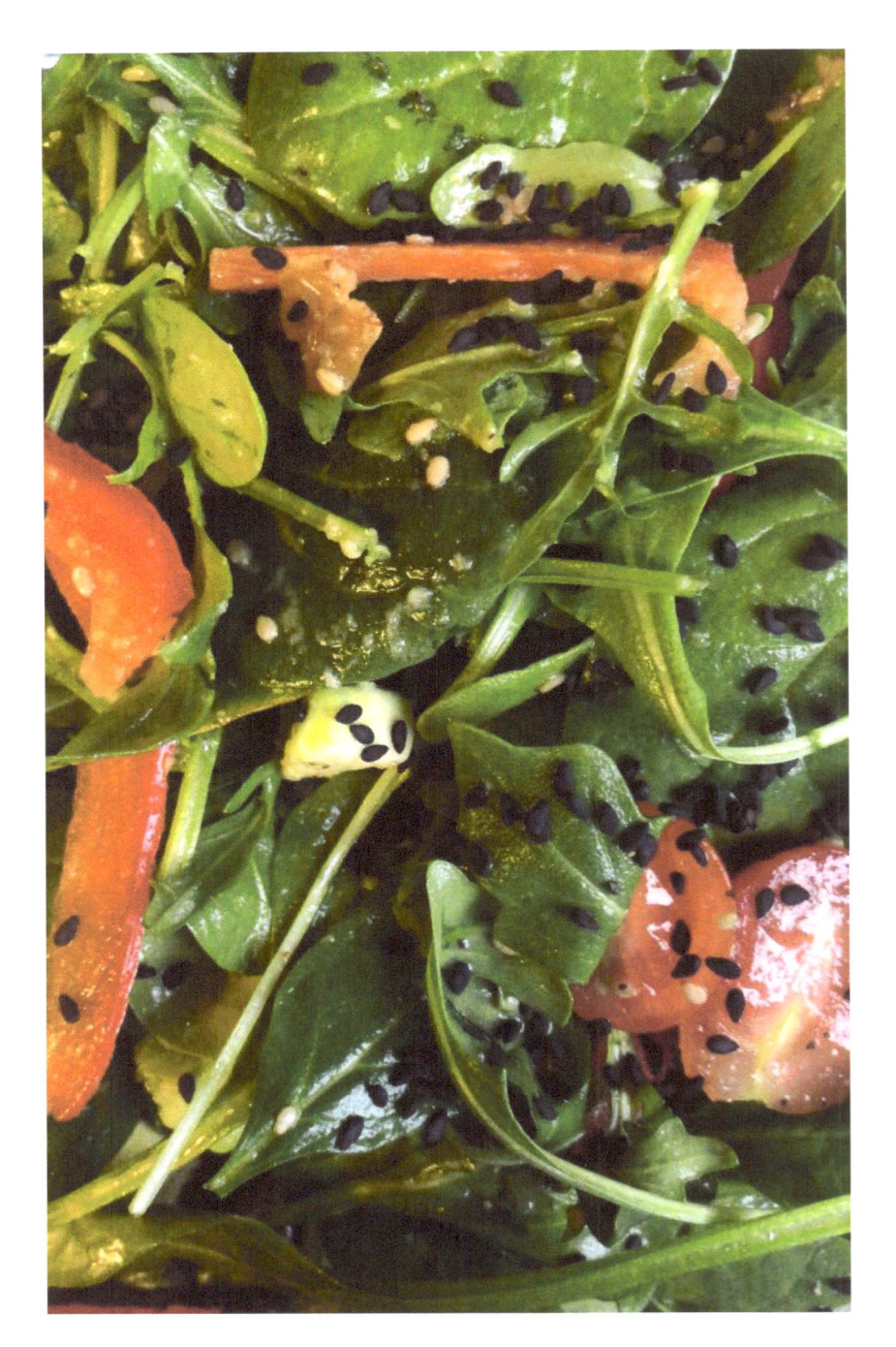

*Photo: Baoku Duduyemi*

Arugula, spinach, avocado, peppers and tomatoes, black and natural/white sesame seeds
Vinaigrette: roasted sesame seed oil, red wine vinegar, salt, pepper

# Lacinato Kale and Swiss Chard Salad

## Baba Baoku

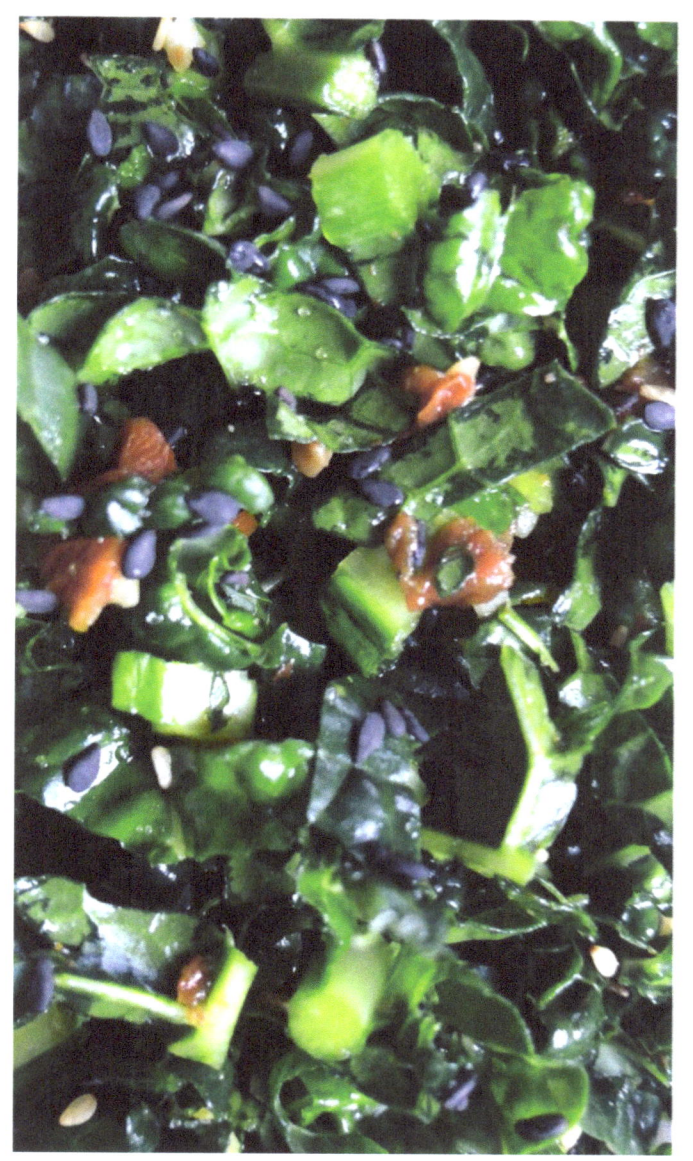

*Photo: Baoku Duduyemi*

## Ingredients:

- 2 bunches of Lacinato kale
- 1 bunch Swiss chard (no stems)
- 5 stems of fresh thyme (leaves only)
- ⅓ cup diced sun-dried tomatoes (soaked)

- 2 tablespoons black sesame seeds
- 1 teaspoon organic natural/white sesame seeds
- 1 tablespoon minced garlic
- 1 tablespoon rich extra virgin olive oil
- 1 tablespoon red wine vinegar
- 1 pinch of Himalayan sea salt

## Directions:

Slice the greens very thinly. Massage all ingredients and serve.

Option: To create a delicious collard green salad, substitute the kale and chard for 2 bunches of organic collard greens sliced very thinly (leaves only). Add ½ red bell pepper (sliced very thinly), and omit the thyme.

# Mama Makes Ends Avocado Salad

## Mama Jasmine

*This was a quick salad I made on a busy Saturday afternoon to feed my hungry boys. They loved it, and so did I! The creaminess of the avocado paired well with the freshness of the butterhead lettuce. Black sesame seeds and hemp hearts added to the liberation of this easy raw vegan salad bowl.*

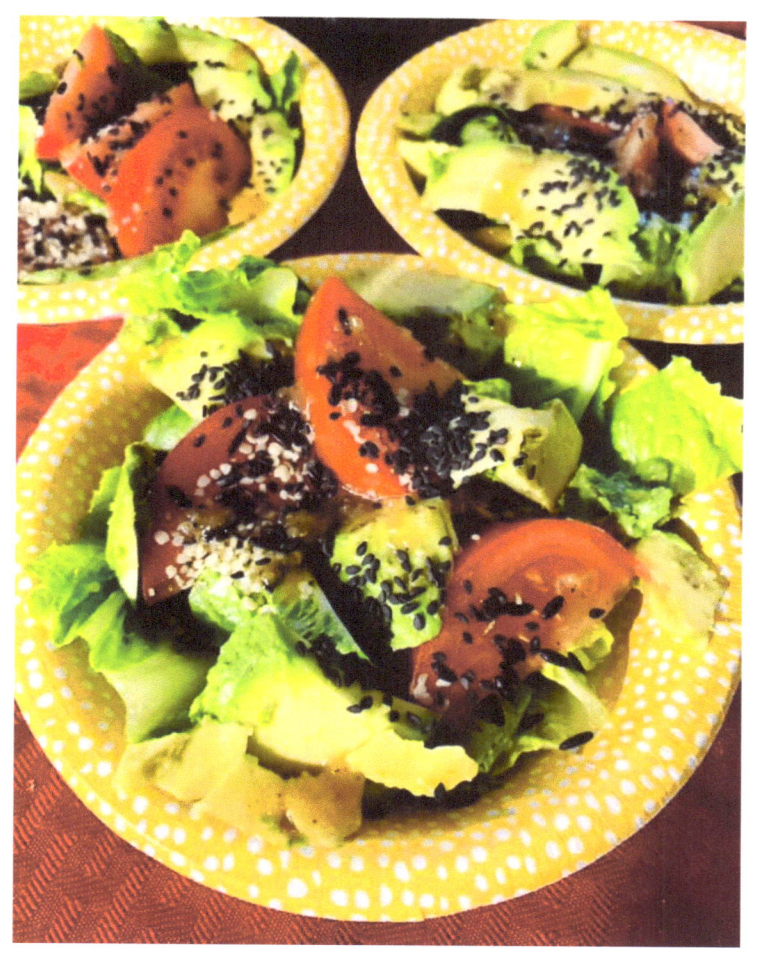

*Photo: Jasmine Barber*

Combine butterhead lettuce, Roma tomatoes, and avocado in a bowl or plate. Sprinkle Braggs 24 Seasoning mix and pink Himalayan salt (optional) to taste. Top with hemp hearts and black sesame seeds. Drizzle with cold-pressed extra virgin olive oil to finish.

# Liberation Kale Salad

## Mama Afiya

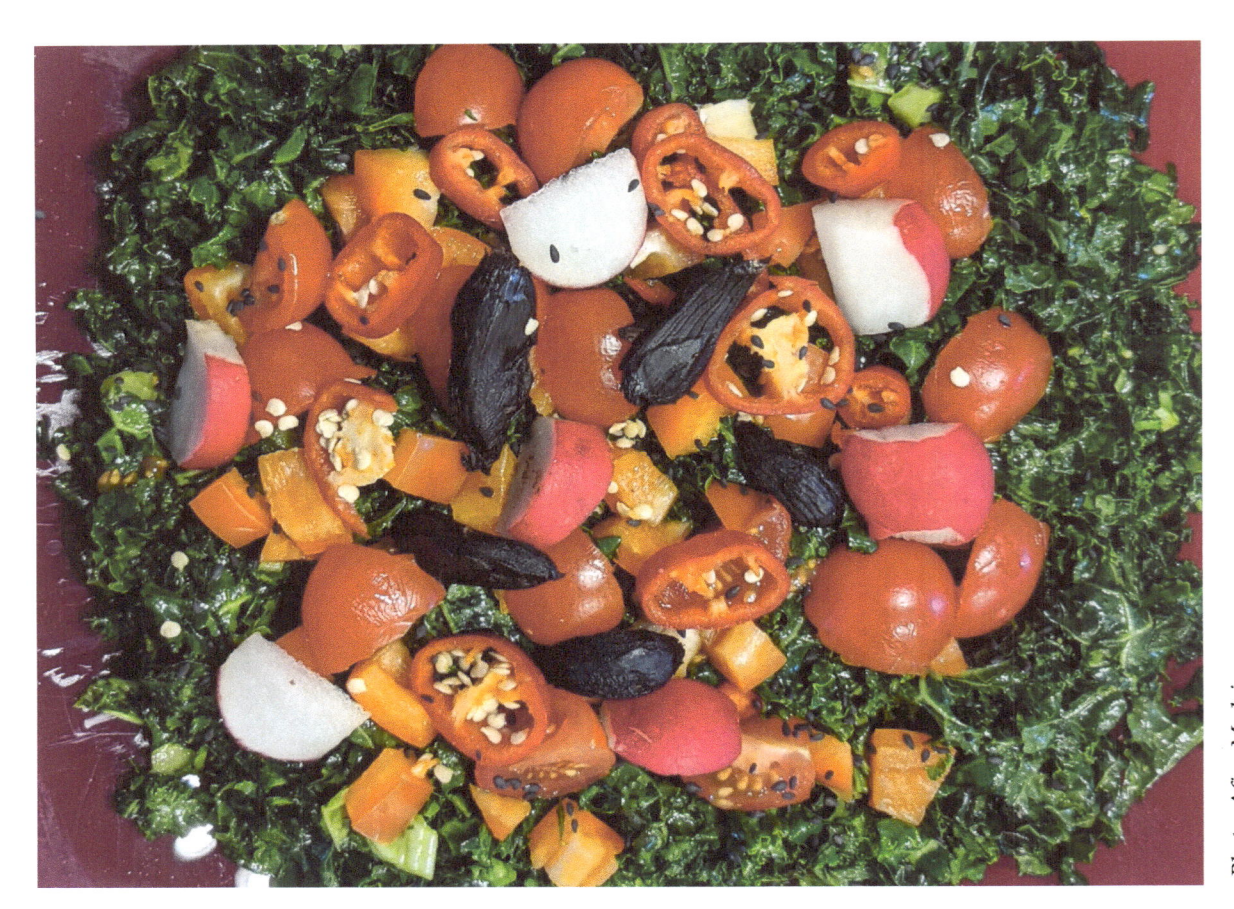

*Photo: Afiya Madzimoyo*

*As we find kale salad sold even at Walmart these days, we are called upon to have a good go-to kale dish much like many of our mamas and grandmamas had their special pot of collard greens. This one always steps up to the occasion -- even when I vary it based upon spontaneous creativity or when I don't have certain staple ingredients on hand.*

## Salad Ingredients:

- 1 large bunch of kale
- A few red tomatoes chopped
- A few sweet red pepper rings
- Small red radish rough sliced
- A few black garlic cloves
- Tahini Dressing Ingredients:
- 1 tablespoon of tahini

- 1 clove of garlic
- ¼ small onion
- 1 tablespoon of chopped fresh ginger
- ½ cup water
- ½ cup nutritional yeast
- 1 teaspoon salt
- 1 teaspoon chickpea miso

## Directions:

Wash and spin kale ahead of time so it is not soggy and will absorb tahini dressing nicely.

Place tahini, garlic, onion, ginger, water, nutritional yeast, salt, and chickpea miso into a blender. Blend until smooth with a consistency to your liking.

Hand massage dressing into the kale.

Arrange red tomatoes, peppers, radishes, and black garlic on top.

# Big Raw Lunch Salad with Butterhead Lettuce and Alfalfa Sprouts

## Mama Jasmine

*This raw vegan salad was so tasty and filling for me during my summer and fall Kemetic Rawer Food Challenge. I could feel myself walking in nutritional power and vibrant self-determination.*

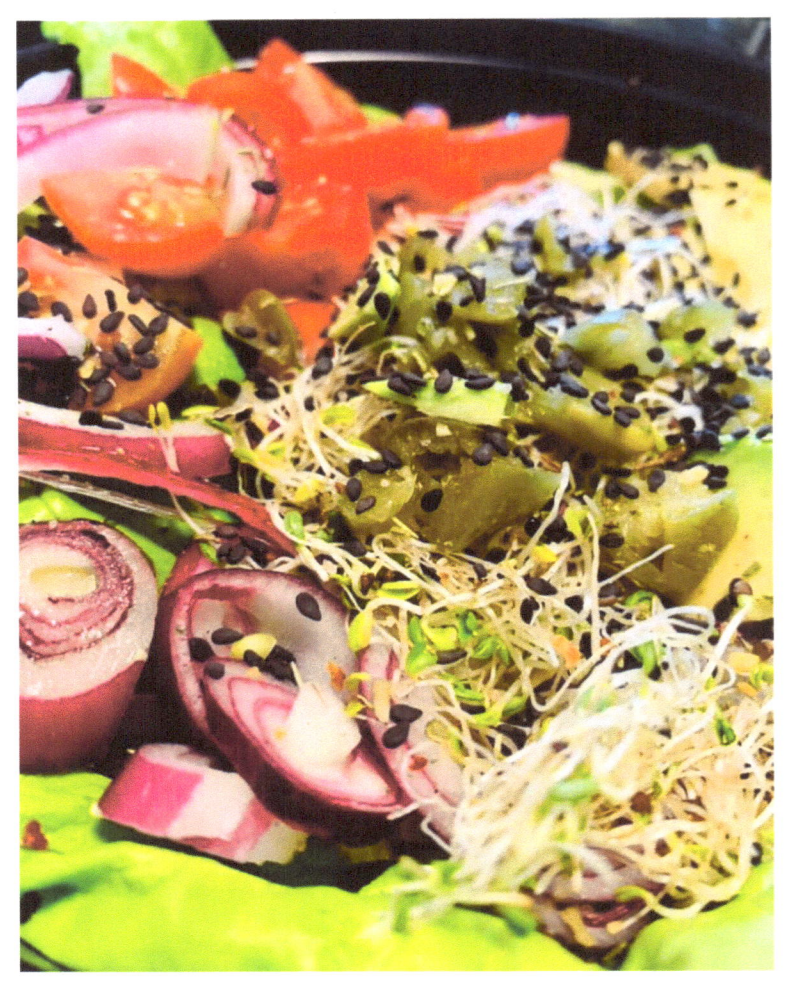

*Photo: Jasmine Barber*

Combine butterhead lettuce, alfalfa sprouts, avocado, jalapeño, tomatoes, red onions, and black sesame seeds in a salad bowl. Sprinkle with Braggs 24 Seasoning Mix and pink Himalayan sea salt (optional) to taste. Finish with cold-pressed extra virgin olive oil.

# Black Goddess Watermelon Avocado Salad

## Mama Jasmine

*This was another favorite of mine during a Summer and Fall Kemetic Rawer Food Challenge. This large fruit salad is energizing, nourishing, refreshing, and filling.*

*Every time I prepare this dish, I feel an affinity towards the Kemetic Goddess, Hetheru. Ancient priestesses of Goddess Hetheru were said to be fruitarians.*

*Goddess Hetheru is the goddess of passionate love, desire, and fierce power. She is the fire-spitting destructive power of light that dispels the blindness of ignorance (African Religion Vol. 5: The Goddess by Dr. Muata Ashby). This salad helps me access my strength as a black woman walking in black power.*

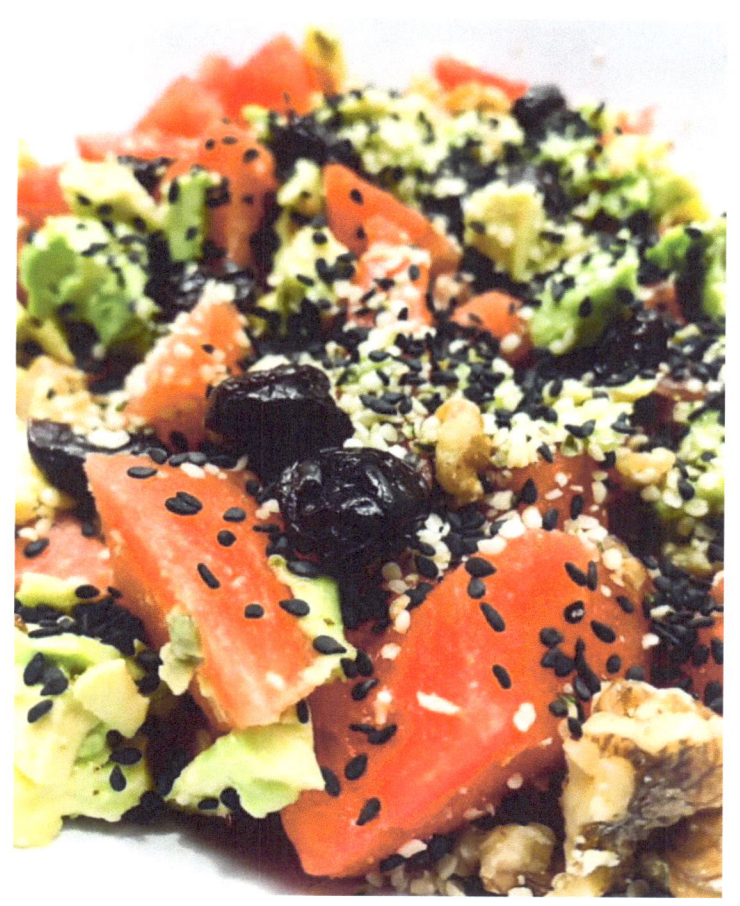

*Photo: Jasmine Barber*

Combine watermelon chunks, avocado slices, tart black cherries, and black walnuts. Top with hemp hearts and black sesame seeds.

# Spring Strawberry Salad

## Mama Johnika

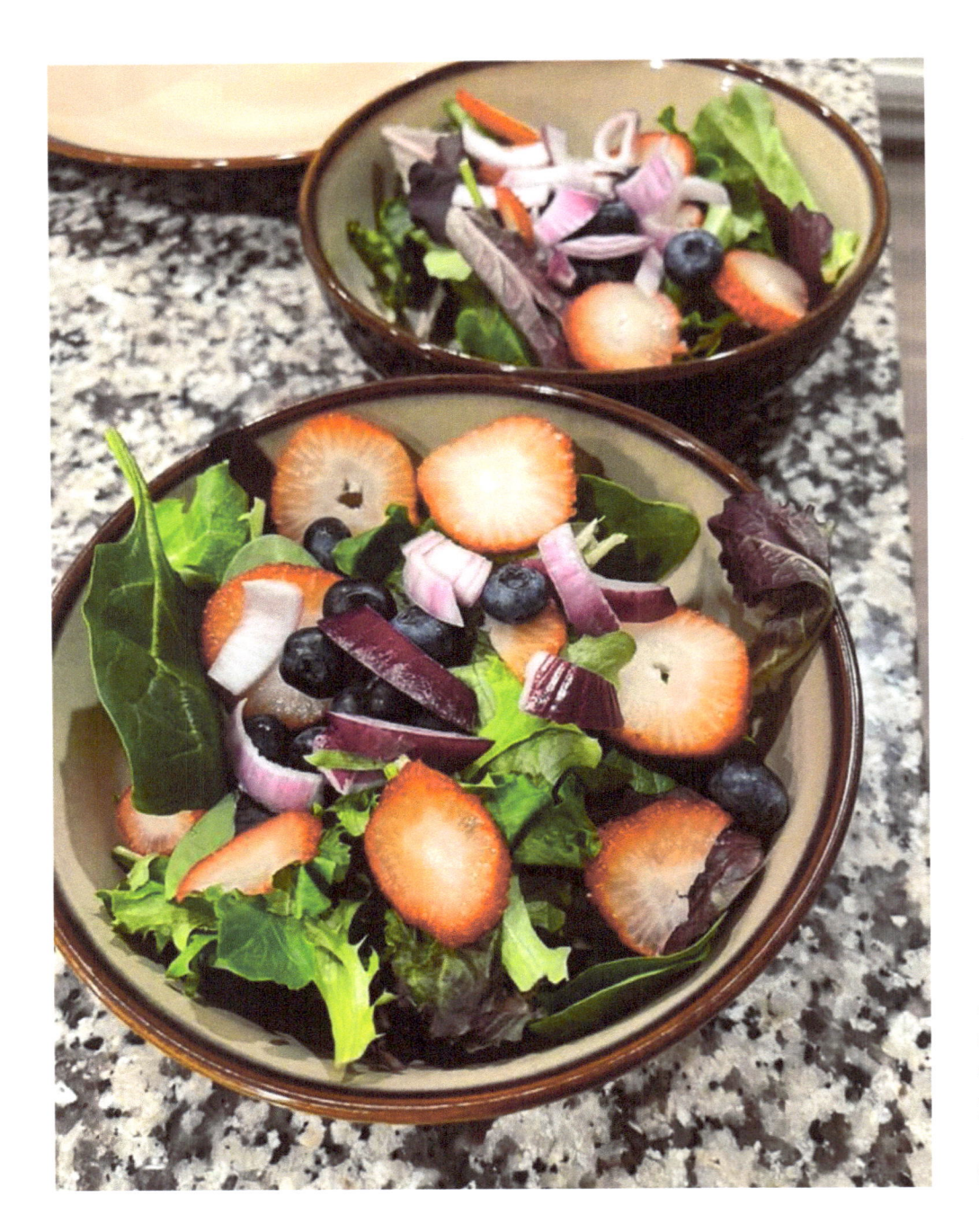

*Photo: Johnika Dreher*

Strawberries, blueberries, red onions, and a strawberry vinaigrette on a bed of leafy greens.

## Ingredients for Strawberry Vinaigrette:

- 8 ounces frozen strawberries
- 2 tablespoons organic, raw honey
- 2 tablespoons apple cider vinegar
- 2 tablespoons olive oil
- ¼ teaspoon salt
- ¼ teaspoon ground black pepper

## Directions:

Blend all ingredients in a blender until smooth. Adjust seasonings to taste.

# *Salad Fruity Nutty Seedy*

## Mama Cheptu

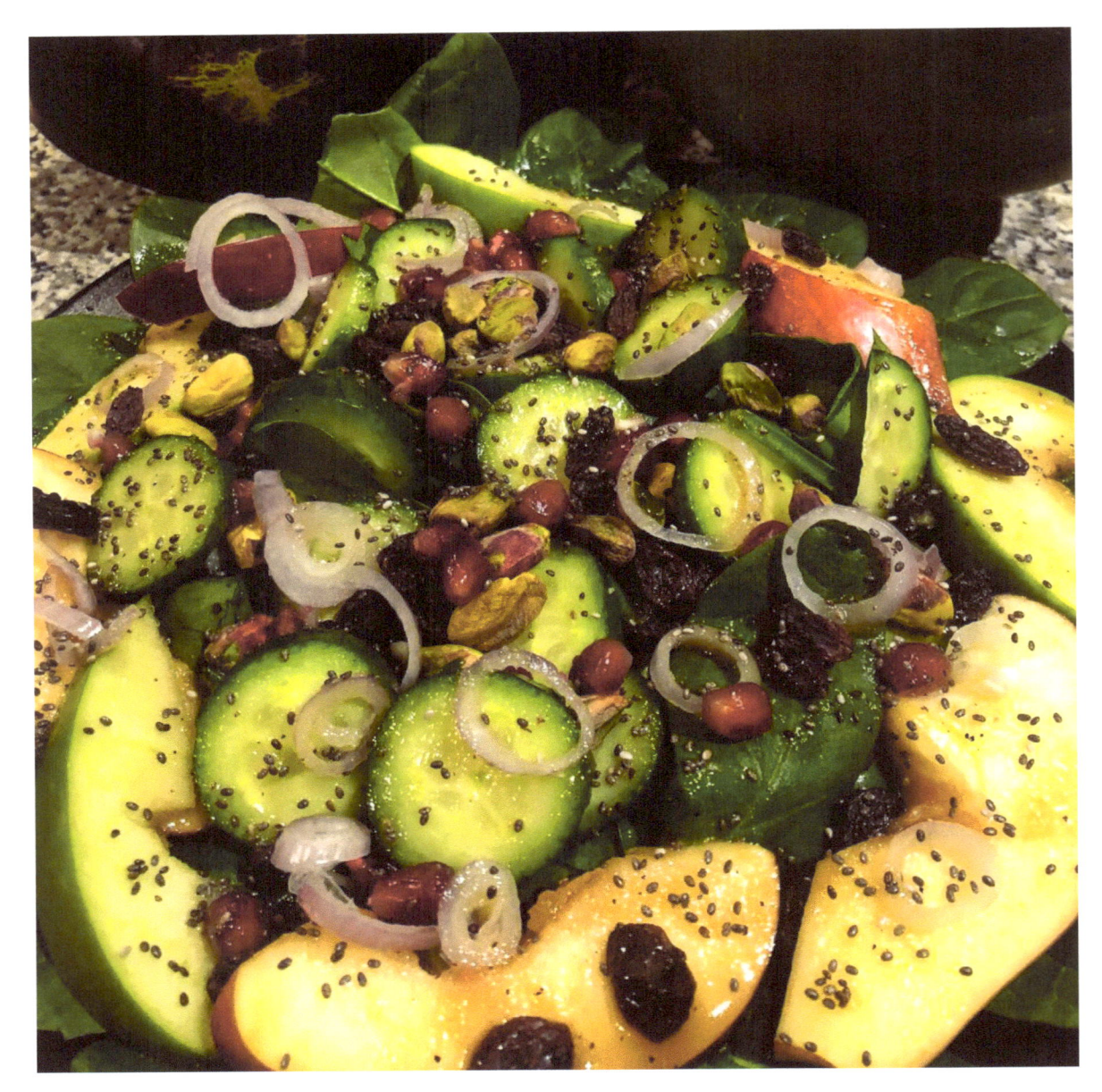

*Photo: Grace Cheptu*

Baby spinach, red and green apples, Persian cucumbers, shallots, raisins, pomegranate seeds, pistachios, pumpkin seeds, black chia seeds, pomegranate vinaigrette

# Pomegranate Vinaigrette

## Ingredients:

- ⅓ cup extra-virgin olive oil
- ⅓ cup pomegranate juice
- ¼ cup red wine vinegar
- 1–2 tablespoons honey or maple syrup, to taste
- 2 teaspoons Dijon mustard
- pinch of salt and pepper

## Directions:

Whisk all ingredients together in a small bowl or shake all together in a sealed jar until evenly combined. Taste and season with extra salt and pepper if needed. Serve immediately or refrigerate in a sealed container for up to one week.

# RBG Fruit Plate

## Mama Khem

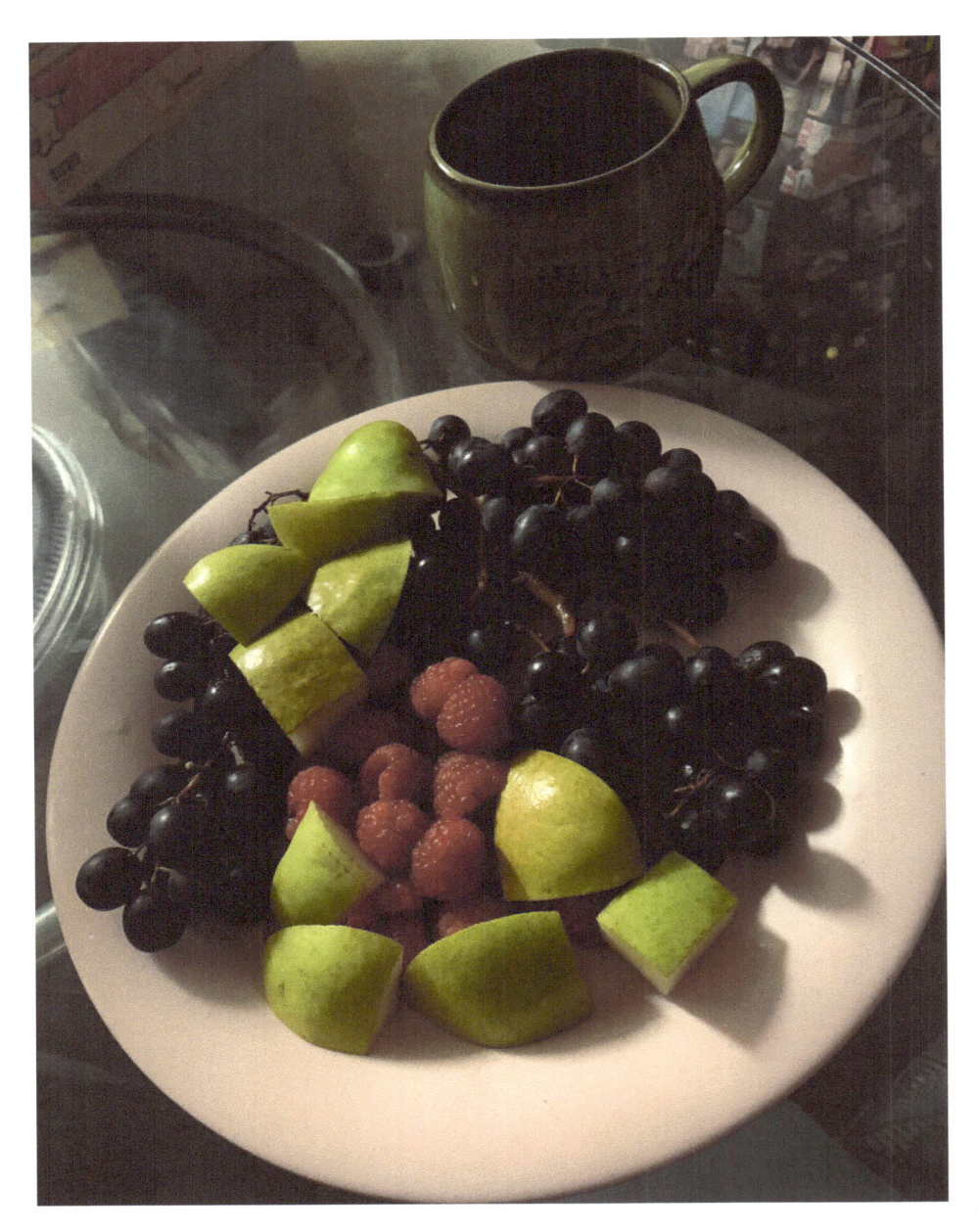

Black grapes, green apples, raspberries

# Red Lentil Soup with Roasted Tomatoes and Red Peppers

## Mama Cheptu

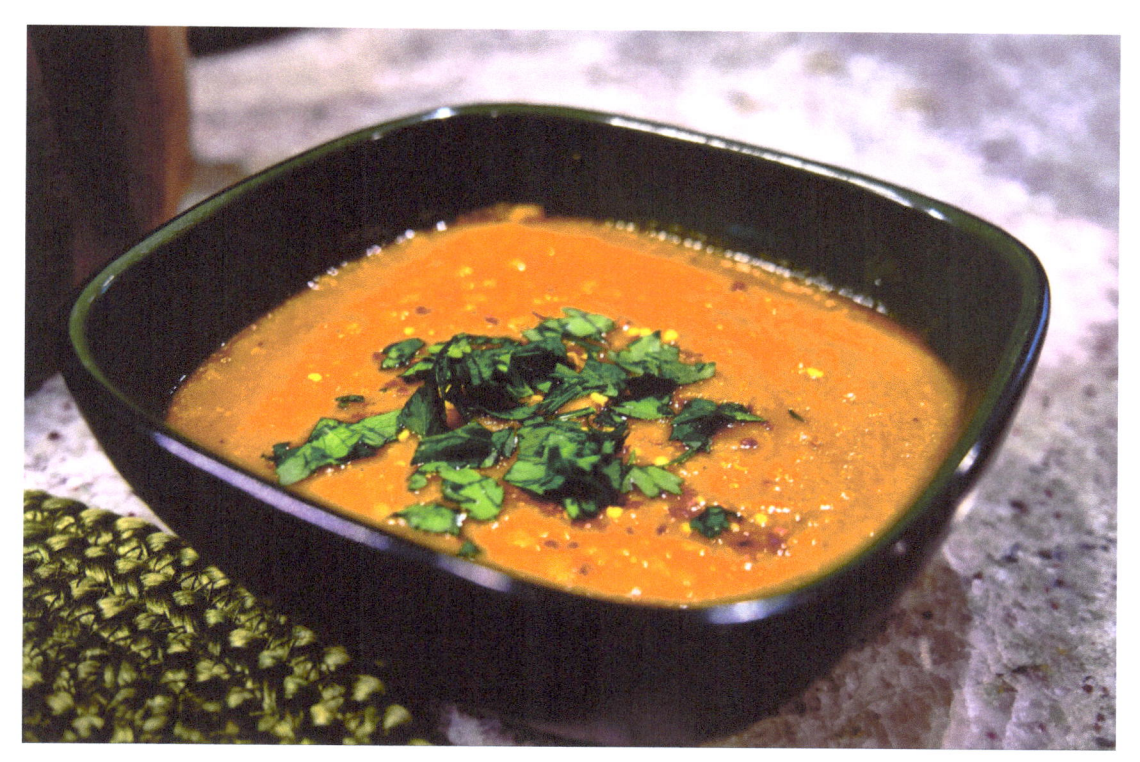

*Photo: Wekesa O. Madzimoyo*

## Ingredients:

- 1½ cups red lentils, picked over and rinsed
- 1 pint cherry tomatoes, halved
- 1 red bell pepper
- 2 large carrots
- 4 cups vegetable broth
- 2 cups coconut water
- 1 tablespoon tomato paste
- 1 large onion, chopped fine
- 1 garlic clove, minced
- 2 tablespoons lemon juice, plus extra for a splash before serving
- 1 tablespoon Harissa Seasoning (North African blend of ground coriander, cumin, ginger, cinnamon, mint, paprika)

- 1 cinnamon stick
- Salt and freshly ground black pepper, to taste
- 4 tablespoons olive oil
- 1 teaspoon paprika
- ¼ cup chopped fresh cilantro

## Directions:

Preheat oven to 450 degrees F. Scrape and slice carrots into ½ inch rounds. Break red bell pepper into large chunks (4-6 pieces). Remove membrane and seeds, then place, along with the tomatoes, into a large bowl with half the olive oil. Coat evenly, then transfer to a flat roasting pan. Roast uncovered for about 20 minutes or until tender. Remove, cool, then process in a blender with one cup of stock. Set aside.

Saute onion and garlic in the remaining olive oil until translucent. Add the harissa seasoning, black pepper, and cook until fragrant, about 2 minutes. Stir in tomato paste and cook another minute. Stir in the blended vegetables, 3 more cups of broth, coconut water, lentils, and cinnamon stick. Cover and simmer for about 15 minutes, occasionally stirring to prevent sticking. When the lentils are soft and mostly broken down, stir vigorously for 30-60 seconds until they are the consistency of a coarse puree. Stir in lemon juice, and adjust salt and pepper to taste. To serve, sprinkle with paprika and garnish with red bell pepper, cilantro, mint, or whatever you like! After a day, this recipe is even better, and it freezes very well.

# Black Bean Soup with Tomatoes and Fresh Spinach

## Mama Cheptu

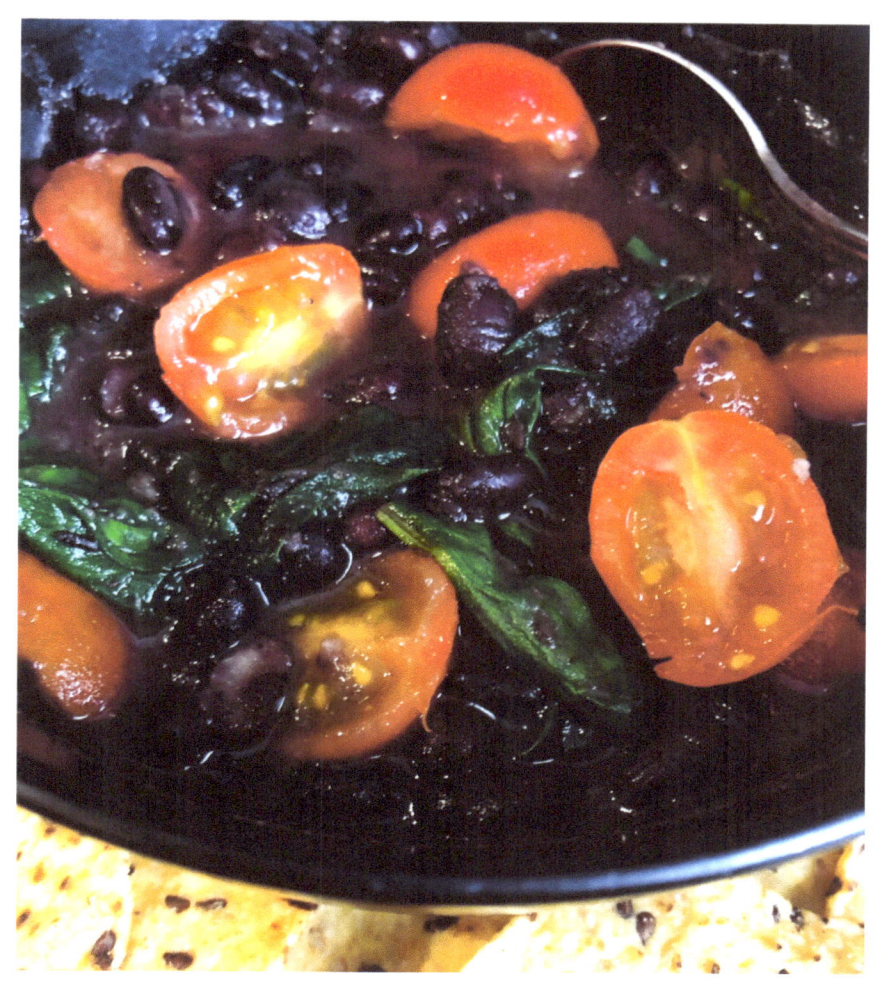

*Photo: Grace Cheptu*

*Oh, gosh, we grew up on beans, beans, beans, and more beans! My mother was thrifty and ensured that we had balanced nutrition, even during financially lean times. She stashed up on dried beans, every kind available. That's pretty much what we ate if local seafood wasn't available or it wasn't our Sunday meat dinner. She always served these dried beans with rice to complete the protein profile. We didn't have access to black beans, but I began to enjoy them when I met Hilda, an elder colleague, on my first job out of college. Hilda was from Cuba, and whenever we'd have potluck celebrations, she'd bring her famous pot of black beans.*
*She got me hooked with her recipe! I've adapted my recipe over the years and now exclusively make them vegan.*

## Ingredients:

- 1 pound bag of organic black beans
- ¼ cup extra virgin olive oil
- 2 quarts vegetable stock or water
- 2 teaspoons smoked sea salt (plain sea salt okay)
- 1 teaspoon freshly ground black pepper
- ½ teaspoon ground oregano
- 1 large bay leaf
- 1 teaspoon ground cumin
- 2 medium jalapeno peppers
- 1 medium head fresh garlic
- 3 large celery stalks
- 1 green bell pepper
- 1 large onion
- ¼ cup lime juice
- ¼ cup roughly chopped cilantro
- Optional toppings: cherry tomatoes, avocado, cilantro, fresh spinach

## Directions:

Rinse the dried black beans in water. Discard any broken, malformed, and or blemished beans. Drain. Replace the water and soak beans overnight. Drain the beans in the morning and discard the water.

Add beans to a large stockpot and cover in freshwater or vegetable stock. Add a bay leaf, salt, freshly ground black pepper, and olive oil. Bring to a boil, then turn down low to simmer, about one hour. While it's simmering, mince your garlic and chop your green bell pepper, onion, celery, and jalapenos. (When I'm in a hurry, I just throw all the fresh veggies in the food processor and keep it moving.) Add the veggies to the pot along with cumin and oregano. Bring to a gentle boil, then turn the heat down to simmer for another hour, or until the beans are tender. They'll eventually get tender, so be patient if it takes longer than an hour. Stir occasionally, so the beans don't stick to the bottom of the pot. Add more water or vegetable stock, if needed.

Once the beans are tender, remove 1 cup of the beans and some of the liquid and process in your blender. Be careful—not too much hot liquid in a blender! Cool it first, or add a couple of ice cubes. Stir the blended mixture back to the pot to create a nicely thickened soup. Adjust seasonings.

Just before serving, stir in the lime juice and chopped cilantro and add your toppings. I added fresh spinach and cherry tomatoes to enhance the liberation look. Top with avocado slices, jalapeno pepper, cilantro, and a slice of lime for a more traditional recipe.

# Snack Time!

## Mama Jasmine

Blue corn and flaxseed tortilla chips with homemade salsa

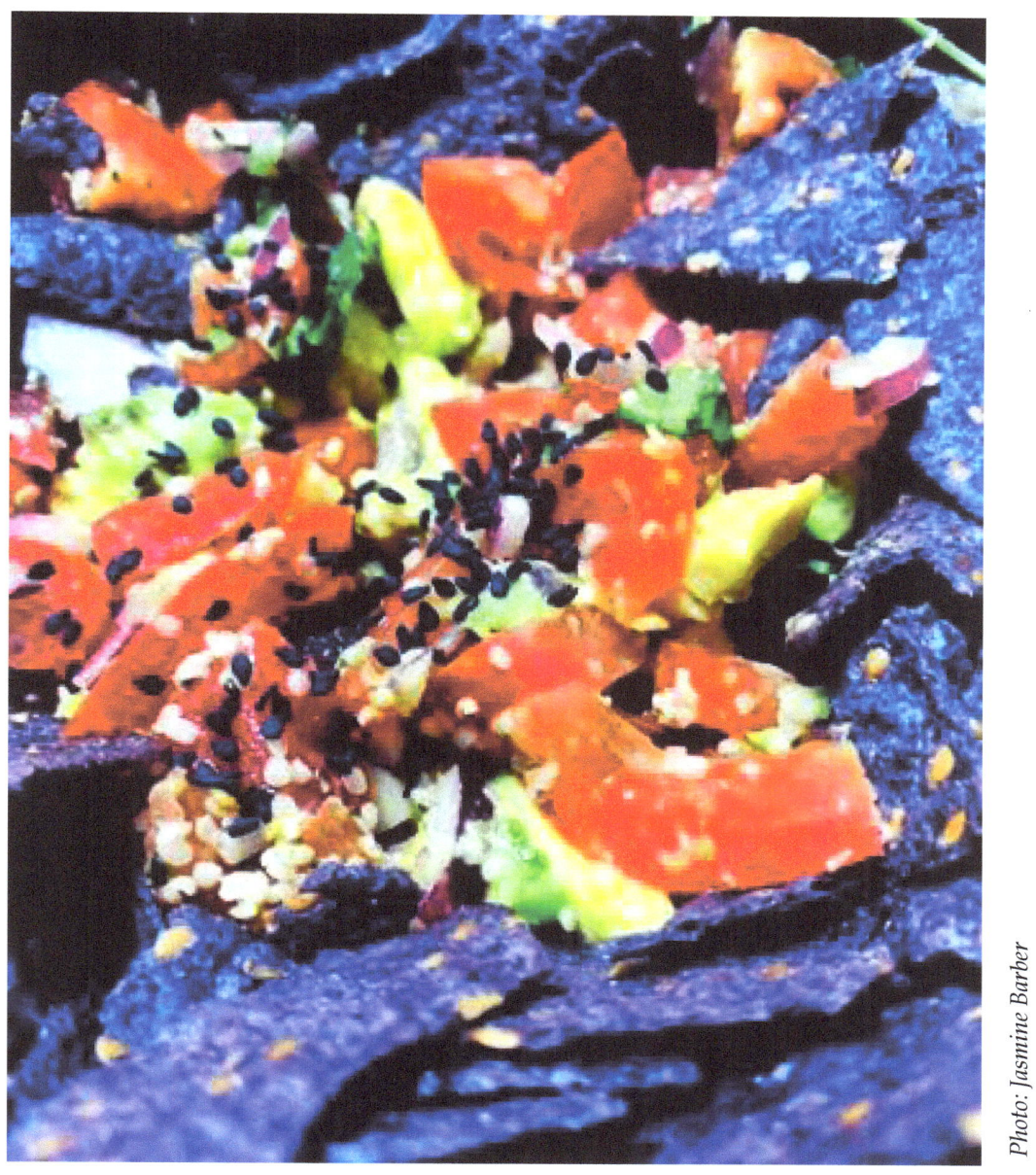

*Photo: Jasmine Barber*

Combine chopped avocado, red onions, cilantro, and tomatoes. Plate with blue corn and flax tortilla chips. Sprinkle with organic hemp hearts and organic black sesame seeds.

# Roasted Veggie Snack

## Mama Cheptu

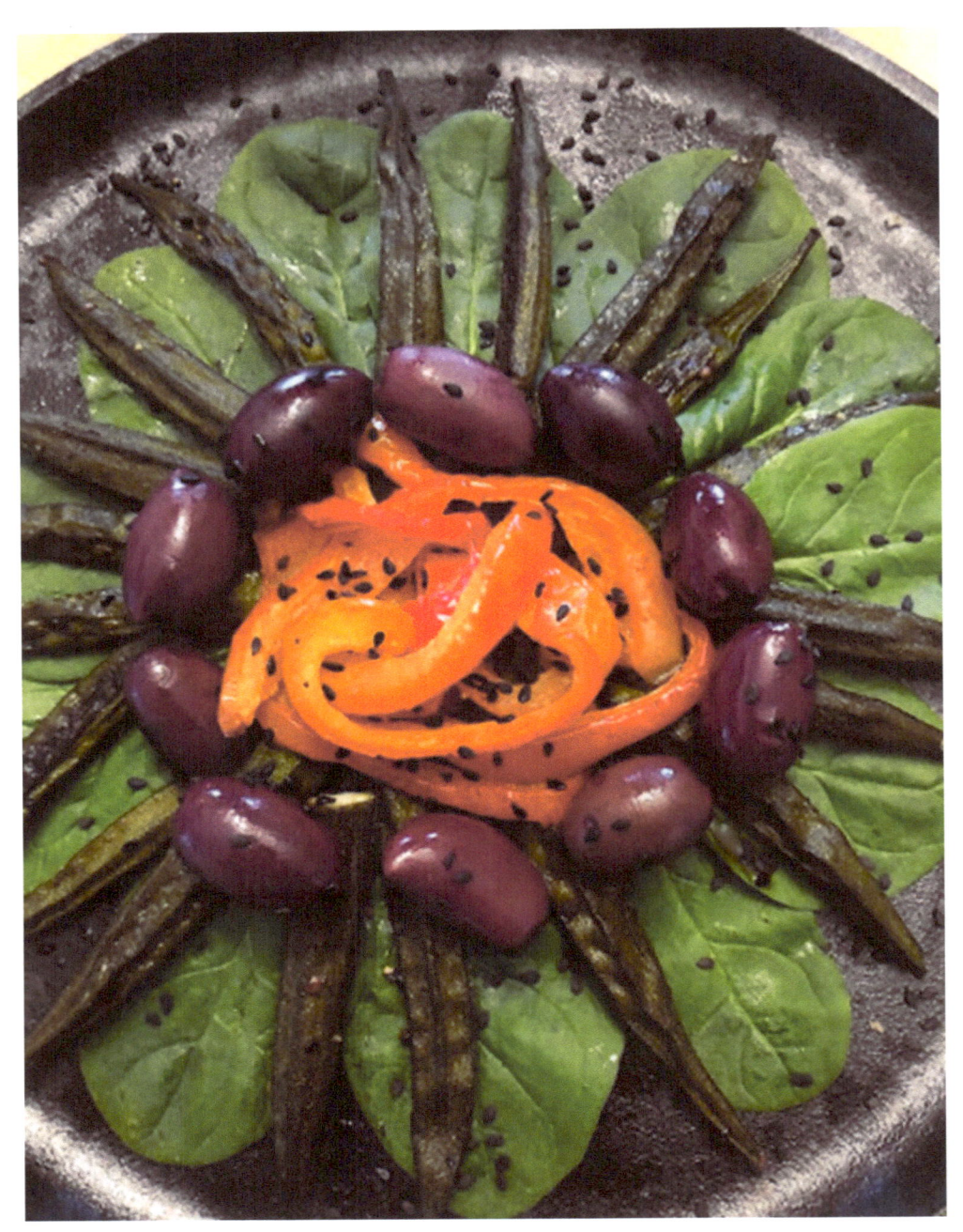

*Photo: Grace Cheptu*

## Ingredients:

- ½ pound okra
- 2 red bell peppers
- 16 or more leaves of spinach
- Kalamata olives
- Black seeds
- 2 tablespoons extra virgin olive oil
- Fresh thyme leaves, optional
- Salt and freshly ground pepper, to taste

## Directions:

Preheat the oven to 450 degrees F. Rinse red pepper and the okra, and dry with a kitchen towel.

Trim away okra stem ends and tips. Place the okra in a large bowl.

After cutting the bell peppers in half, remove the membrane and seeds. Now add the peppers to the bowl of okra. Lightly salt okra and bell peppers and toss with the olive oil until coated.

Lift the okra and peppers out of the oil and spread in a single layer on a sheet pan lined with parchment paper. Roast in the oven for 15 minutes. Gently shake the pan every five minutes.

Remove from the oven. The okra will be lightly seared with a beautiful aroma and not soggy or slimy. The pepper skins will be charred.

When the peppers cool enough to touch, peel away the skin and slice into strips.

Arrange fresh baby spinach leaves on a flat dish. Arrange okra, olives, and red peppers on top and sprinkle with fresh thyme, a little black pepper, and black seeds.

# Fruit-Nut-Seed Snack

## Mama Cheptu

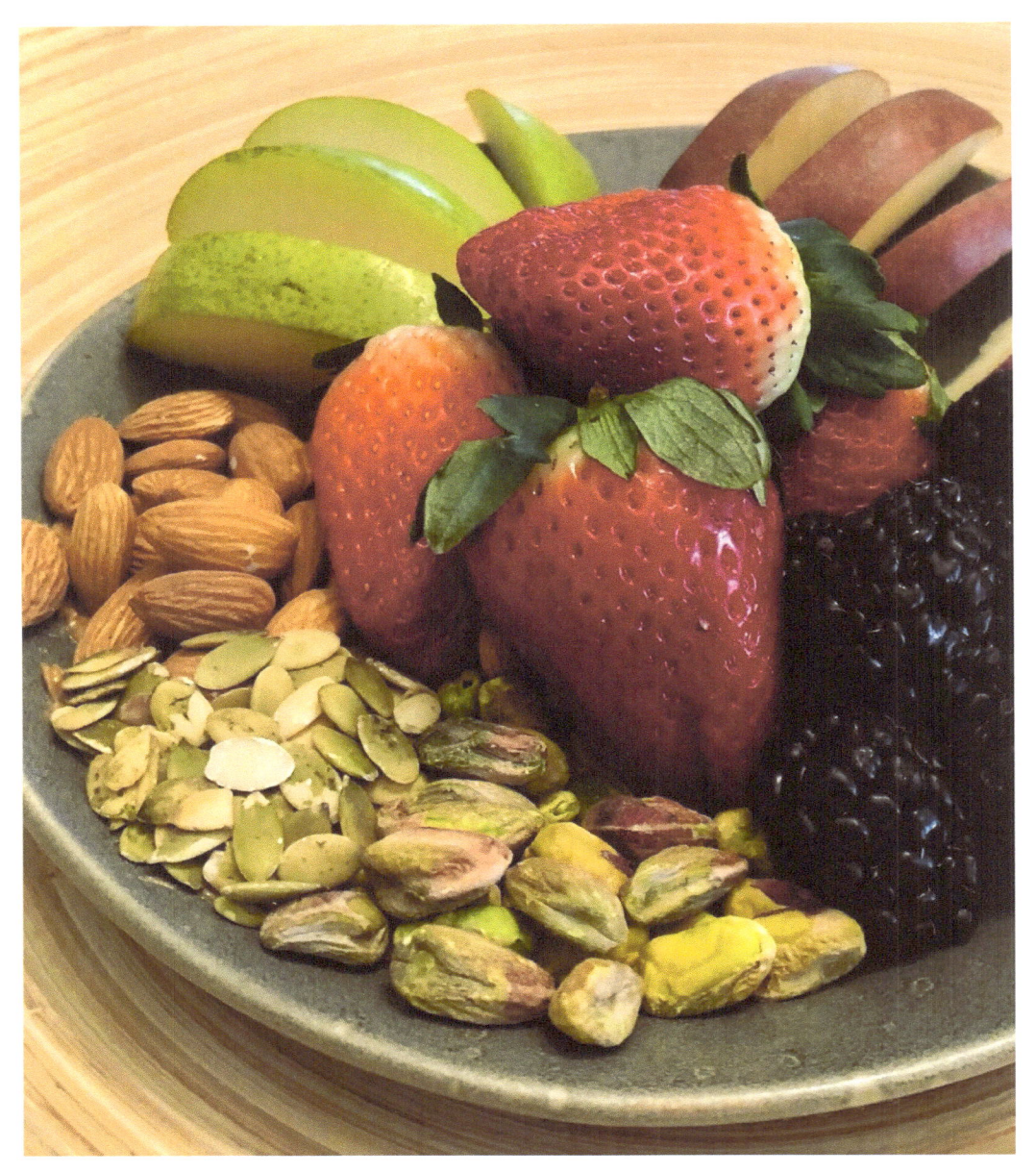

*Photo: Grace Cheptu*

**RED** strawberries and red pear
**BLACK** berries
**GREEN** pistachios, pumpkin seeds, and green pear
with almonds

# Section III: Allomelanins on Deck

## Baba Wekesa

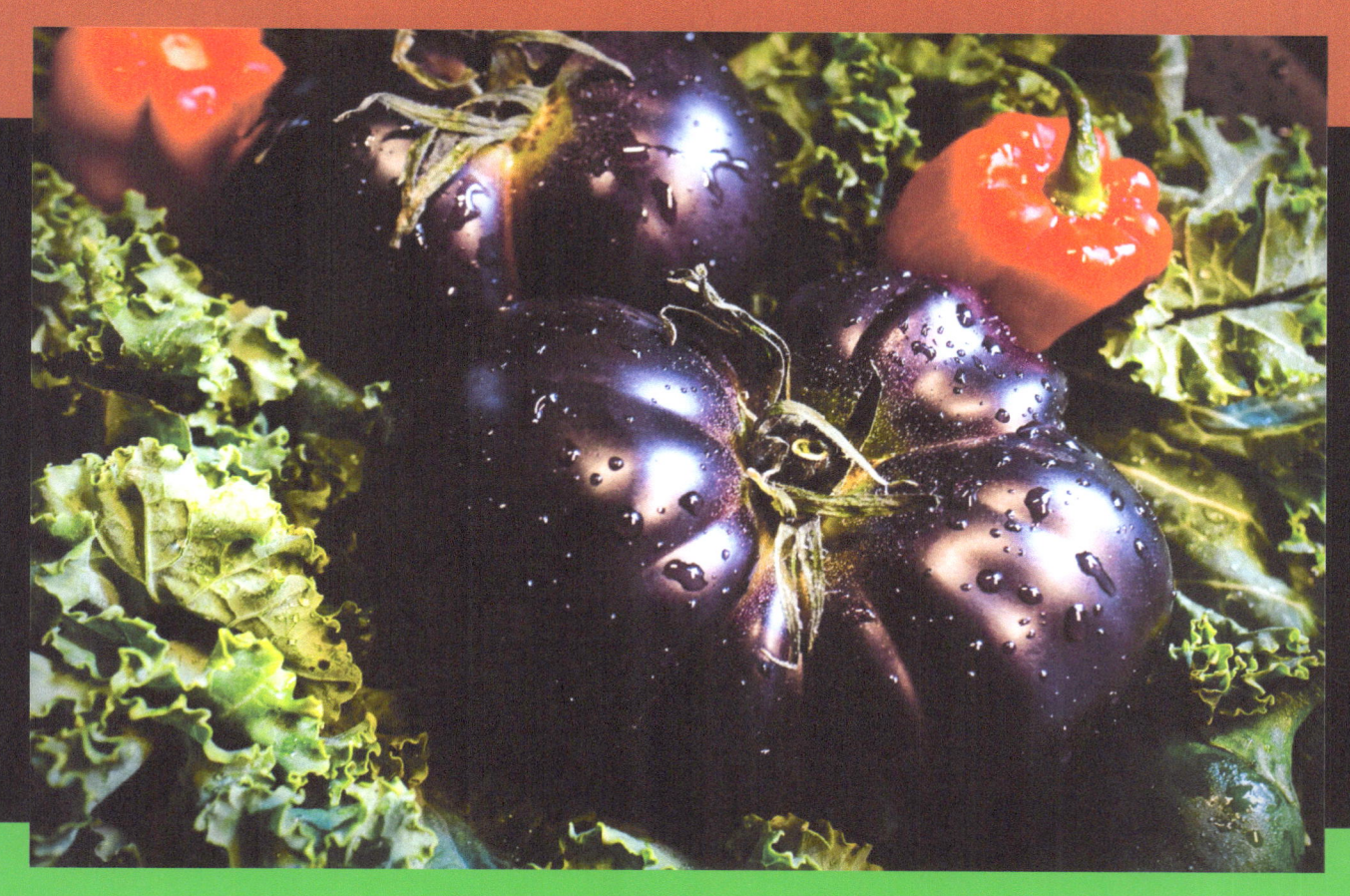

*Photo: Wekesa O. Madzimoyo*

Black garlic, black rice, and black seeds are all allomelanins. Now, add black tomatoes to your list. Black tomatoes have a much higher anthocyanin content because of their purplish or black skin color. Anthocyanins are strong pigments with antioxidant properties whose purpose is to protect plants from ultraviolet radiation from the sun. A diet consisting of foods rich in these pigments bestow the same antioxidant effects and reduce damage produced by harmful reactive oxygen molecules called free radicals.

# Black Rice/Forbidden Rice

## (Orzya sativa L.)

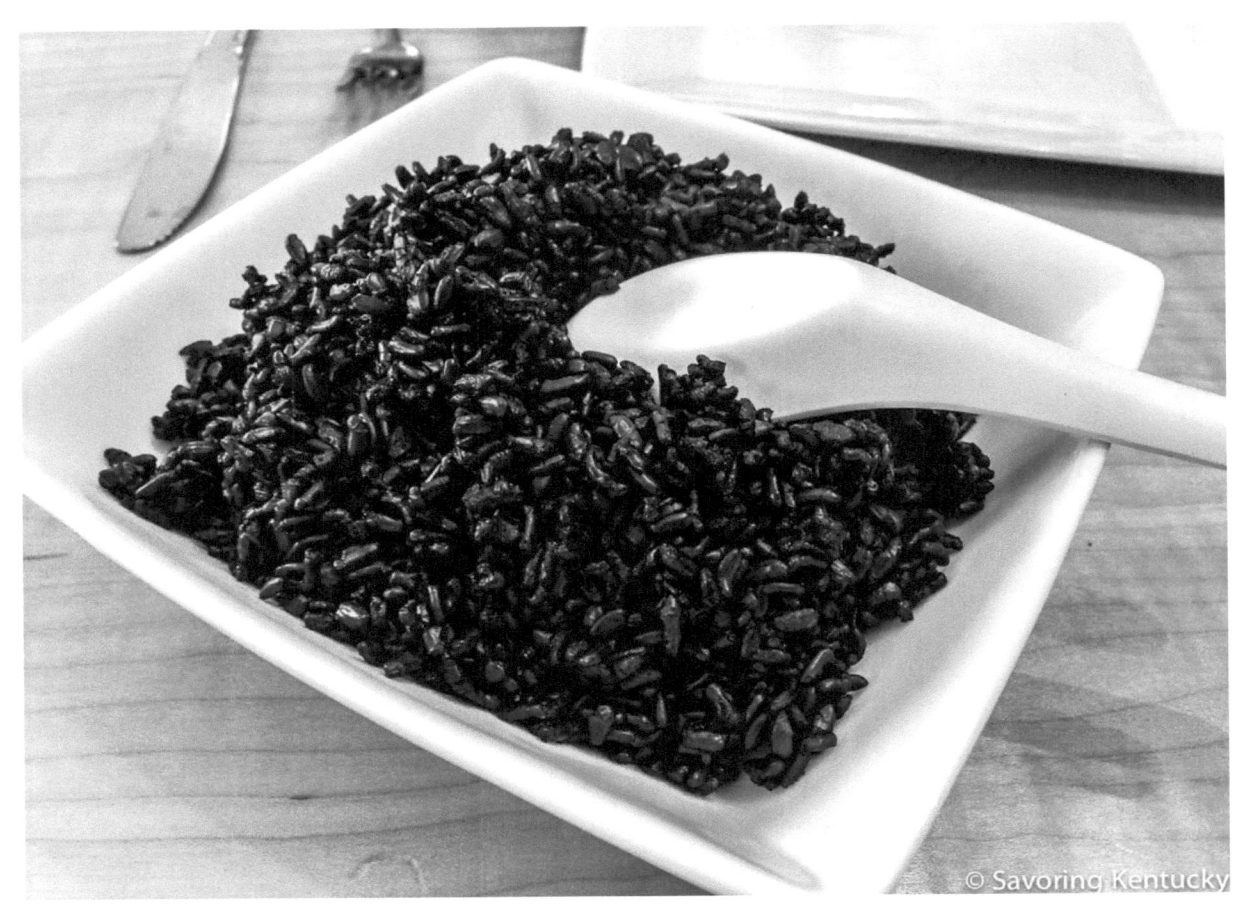

*Photos: "Black rice, white dish" by ronanue licensed under CC BY 2.0.*

Black rice is also called purple rice, heaven rice, imperial rice, king's rice, and prized rice. This heirloom whole food has its origin in ancient China.

Contains higher levels of vitamins, minerals, and proteins than white rice
Rich in the essential amino acids lysine and tryptophan
High source of anthocyanin
Highest antioxidants and dietary fiber of all rice varieties
More antioxidants than blueberries
Enhances health and longevity
Protects heart health
Reduces atherosclerosis
Improves digestive system

Detoxifies the body
Reduces risk of diabetes
Reduces cancer growth
Boosts cognitive function
Rich in vitamins and minerals:
Vitamin B1, Vitamin B2, folic acid, iron, zinc, calcium, phosphorus, selenium

Sources:

Kushwaha, Ujjawal. (2016). Black Rice Research, History and Development. 10.1007/978-3-319-30153-2.

Thanuja B, Parimalavalli R. Role of black rice in health and diseases. Int J Health Sci Res. 2018; 8(2):241-248.

# Black Garlic

## by Baba Wekesa

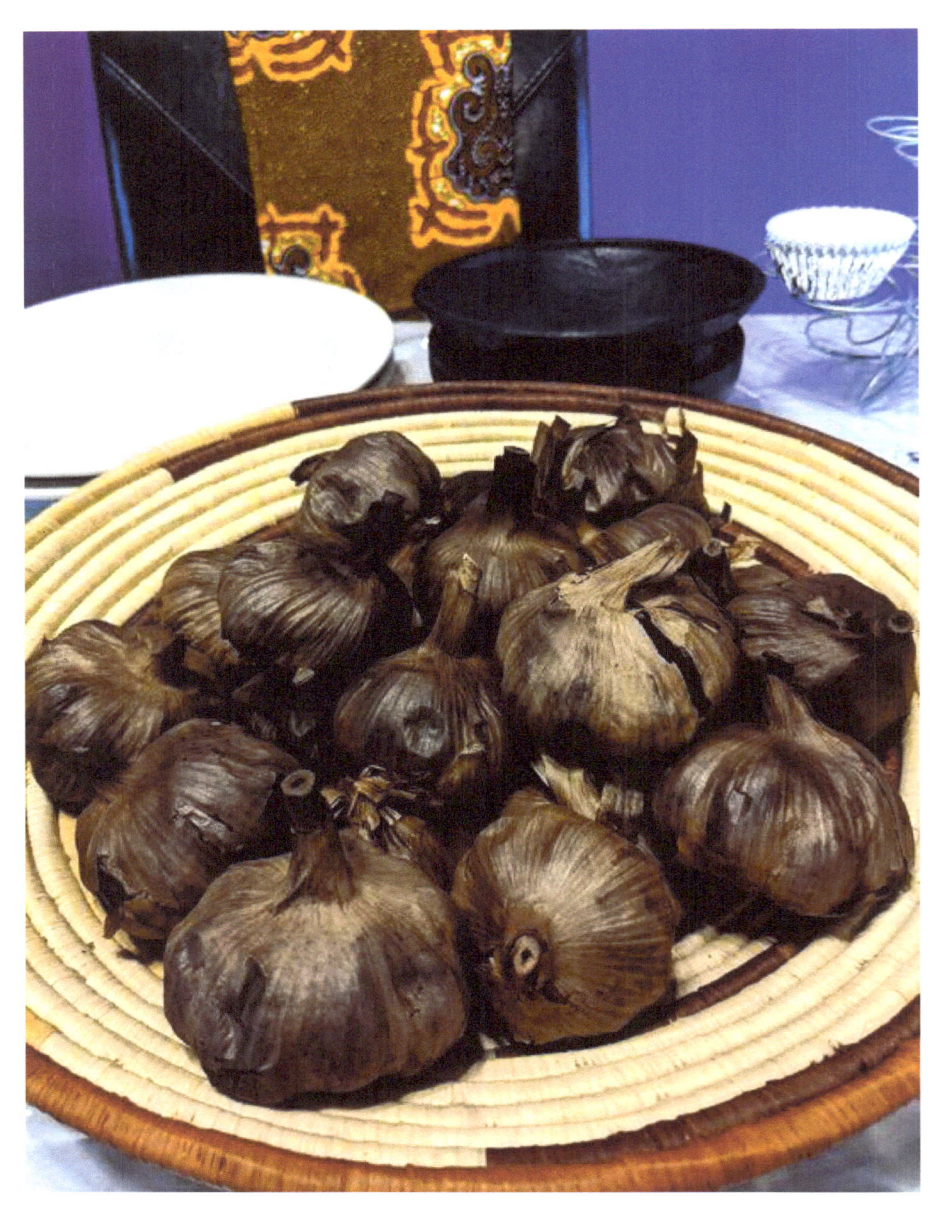

*Photo: Afiya Madzimoyo*

Black garlic anyone?

While black garlic has less of the active compound allicin than its fresh raw counterpart, it does boast higher concentrations of many nutrients, antioxidants, and other beneficial compounds. These higher concentrations may be partly responsible for the many health benefits that black garlic provides:

**Blood Sugar Control**

Like fresh raw garlic, black garlic can help regulate blood sugar levels. Reducing high blood sugar helps prevent serious health issues such as diabetes symptoms, kidney dysfunction, and more. Higher antioxidant levels in black garlic may also prevent complications related to diabetes.

**Heart Protection**

Fresh raw garlic is known for its ability to help improve heart health. Black garlic may provide the same protective effects. Black garlic can also help lower cholesterol and triglycerides, which reduces your risk of heart disease.

**Fights some Cancers**

Many studies show that black garlic's antioxidant properties can help fight against cancer. One study found that it could help reduce the growth of colon cancer cells. Compounds in aged black garlic can also block free radicals in the body. This property reduces cell damage and can help to limit the growth and potential spread of cancer cells in the body.

# Black Sesame Seeds

## (Sesamum radiatum)

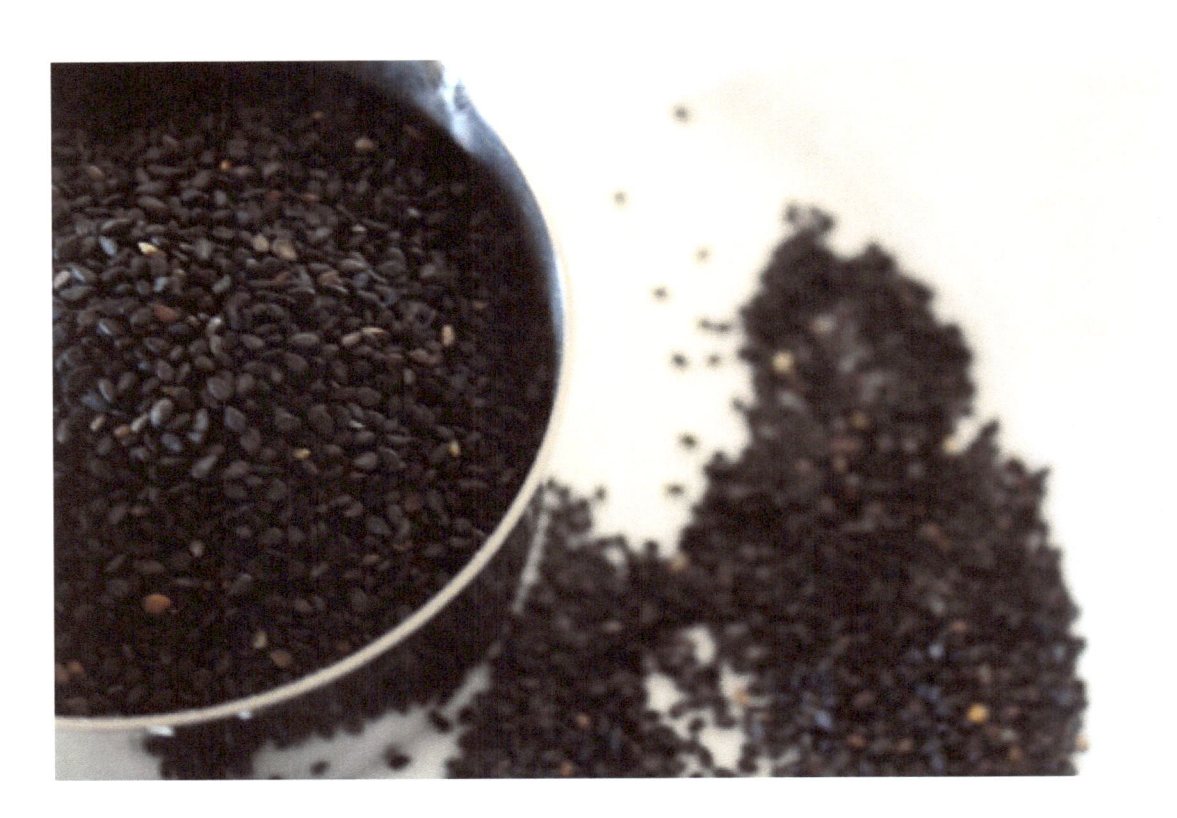

*Photo: "black-sesame-seeds" by WELLinLA licensed under CC BY-NC 2.0*

An ancient oil crop with a long history of more than 2200 years of cultivation

Protects cardiovascular function
May prevent atherosclerosis
Reduces total cholesterol
Protective against chronic liver injury
Antioxidant
Anti-inflammatory
Anti-tumor; anti-cancer
Anti-aging
Protects against neurodegeneration
Decreases antioxidant stress
Prevents osteoporosis
Protective effect in kidneys

Source:

Wang, D., Zhang, L., Huang, X., Wang, X., Yang, R., Mao, J., Wang, X., Wang, X., Zhang, Q., & Li, P. (2018). Identification of Nutritional Components in Black Sesame Determined by Widely Targeted Metabolomics and Traditional Chinese Medicines. Molecules (Basel, Switzerland), 23(5), 1180. https://doi.org/10.3390/molecules23051180.

# Black Seed Oil/Kalonji

## (Nigella sativa)

*Photo: "A Spoon with Black Cumin - Nigella Sativa" by philipp.alexander.ernst licensed under CC BY 2.0*

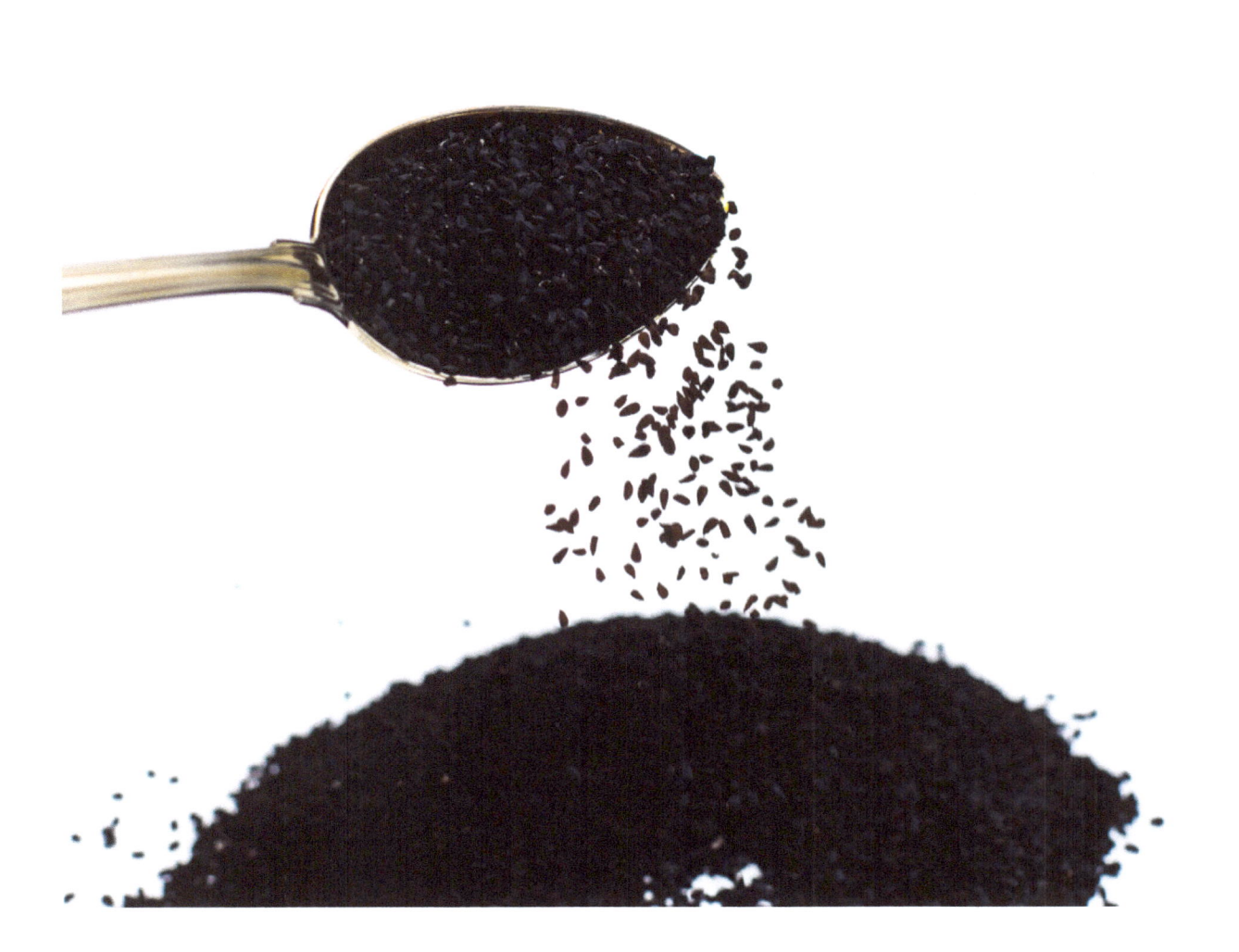

Black seed oil is an ancient healing oil from black cumin seeds. Its uses go back more than 2000 years to African, Indian, and Arabian civilizations as food and medicine.

Rich source of thymoquinone (TQ)
Anti-inflammatory
Anti-microbial
Anti-nociceptive
Anti-epileptic

Anti-cancer for blood, breast, colon, pancreatic, liver, lung, fibrosarcoma, prostate, cervix

Healing for the:
Respiratory system
Digestive tract
Kidney and liver
Cardiovascular system
Immune system

Has cured: hypertension, dyslipidemia, metabolic syndrome, diabetes, asthma, convulsion, natural and chemical toxicities

Great for overall general well-being
Rich in alkaloids, saponins, flavonoids, proteins, fatty acids

Source:

Tavakkoli, A., Mahdian, V., Razavi, B. M., & Hosseinzadeh, H. (2017). Review on Clinical Trials of Black Seed (Nigella sativa ) and Its Active Constituent, Thymoquinone. Journal of pharmacopuncture, 20(3), 179–193. https://www.ncbi.nlm.nih.gov/pmc/articles/PMC5633670/

# Purple Sweet Potato

## (Ipomoea batatas L cultivar Ayamurasaki)

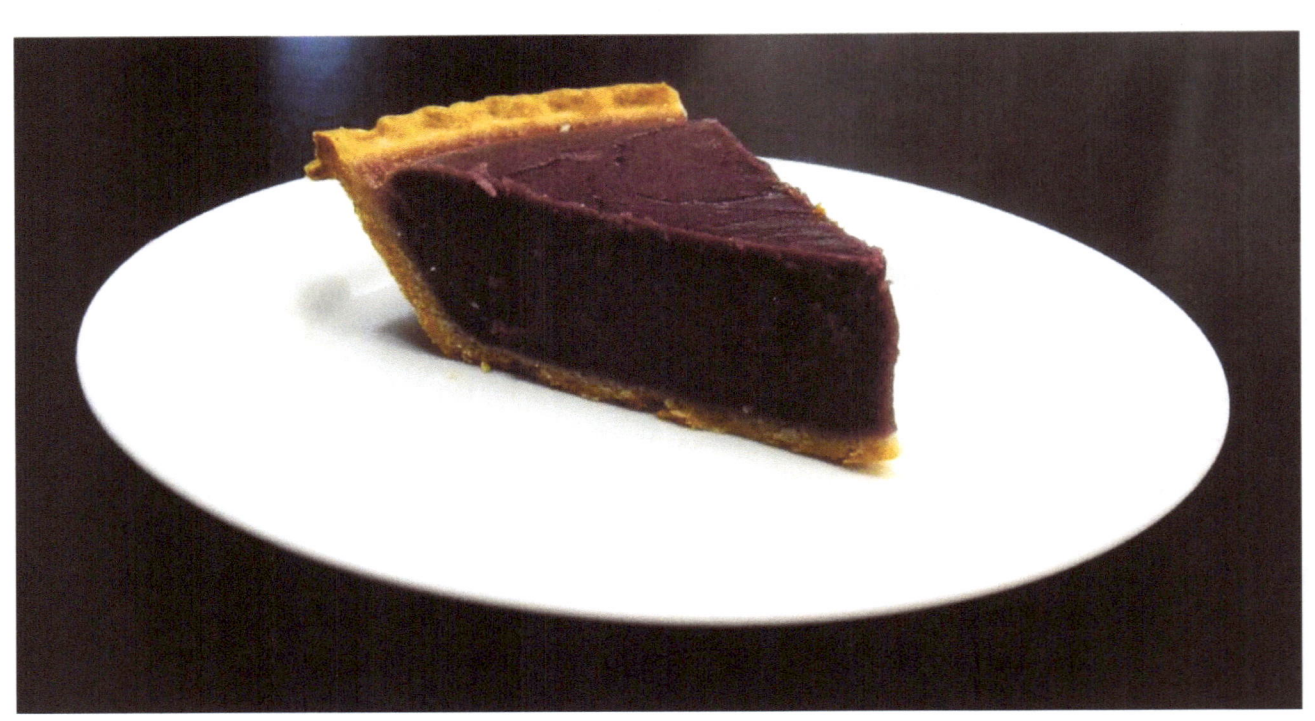

*"Purple Sweet Potato Pie" by arnold | inuyaki licensed under CC BY 2.0*

Purple sweet potatoes are a good source of beta-carotene. They are an even richer source of anthocyanin pigments, which act as antioxidants that can help reduce inflammation and boost your immune system. Purple sweet potatoes have about three times more anthocyanins than the average blueberry.

Health benefits:

Assists in weight loss
Lowers blood pressure
Boosts cognitive function
Improves digestive health
Prevents gout
Improves liver health
Slows down the aging process
Manages symptoms of diabetes
Anti-cancer properties

Source:

Li A, Xiao R, He S, An X, He Y, Wang C, Yin S, Wang B, Shi X, He J. Research Advances of Purple Sweet Potato Anthocyanins: Extraction, Identification, Stability, Bioactivity, Application, and Biotransformation. Molecules. 2019 Oct 23;24(21):3816. doi: 10.3390/molecules24213816. PMID: 31652733; PMCID: PMC6864833.

# Black Tomatoes

## (Solanum chilense, S. hirsutum, S. cheesmanii, and S. lycopersicoides)

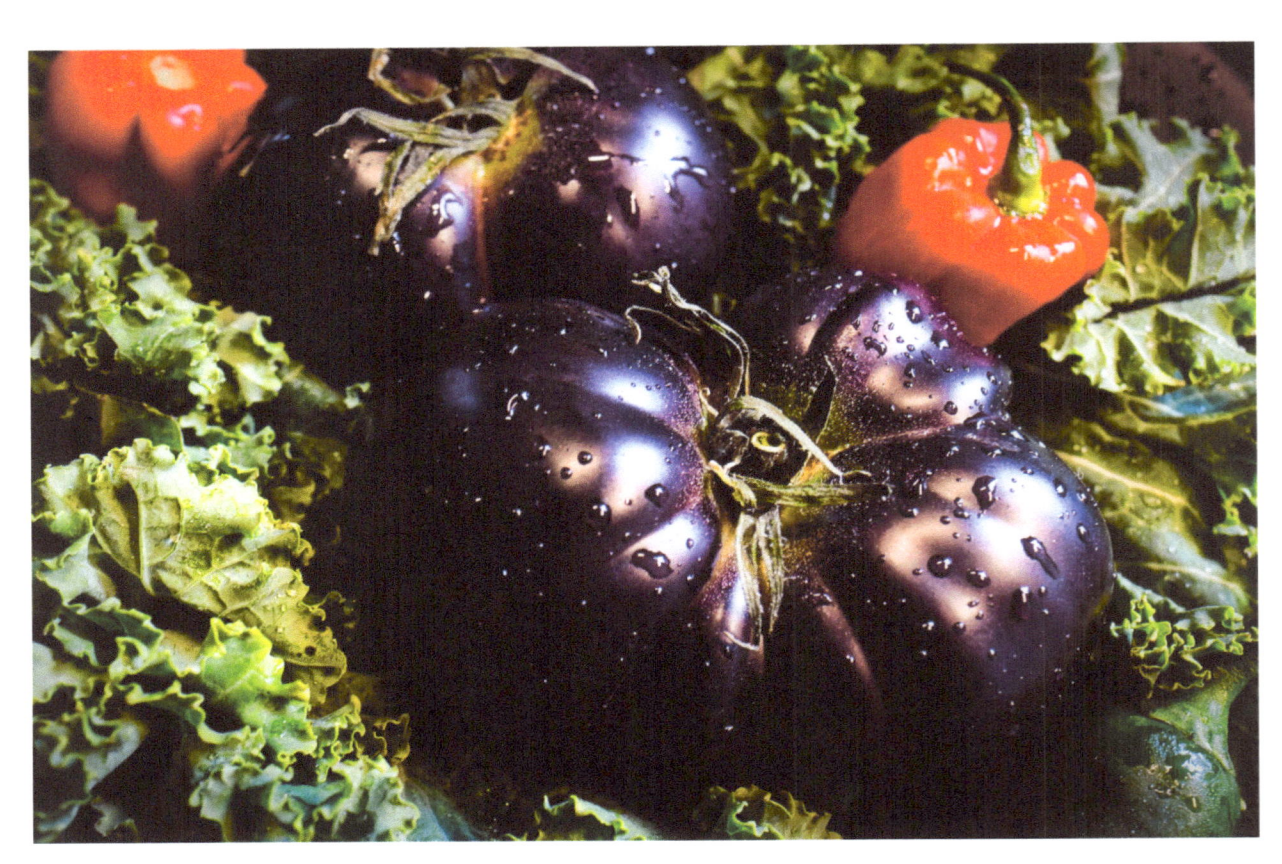

*Photo: Wekesa O. Madzimoyo*

This Ngolo Garden summertime favorite is a rich source of carotenoids and flavonoids (especially flavonols and flavones). Ingesting the black tomato seeds increases circulating melatonin levels in the body for sleep support.

High source of lycopene, beta carotene, vitamin C, and hydroxycinnamic acid
Anti-inflammatory
Anti-proliferative
Anti-cancer properties
Boosts sperm production
Prevents cardiovascular diseases
Helps with sleep management
Improves fertility disorders
Protective against diabetes, and chronic degenerative diseases
Improves cognitive performance and function

Source:

Perna, Simone & Tawfik, Sherry & Alalwan, Tariq & Gasparri, Clara & Peroni, Gabriella & Alaali, Zahraa & Mubarak, Hind & Butti, Ebtisam & Infantino, Vittoria & Rondanelli, Mariangela. (2020). Bioactives Profile of Purple and Black Tomato: Potential Applications in the Pharmaceutical Field Purple and Black Tomato. Indian Journal of Pharmaceutical Sciences. 82. 10.36468/pharmaceutical-sciences.724.

# Saw Palmetto

## (Serenoa repens)

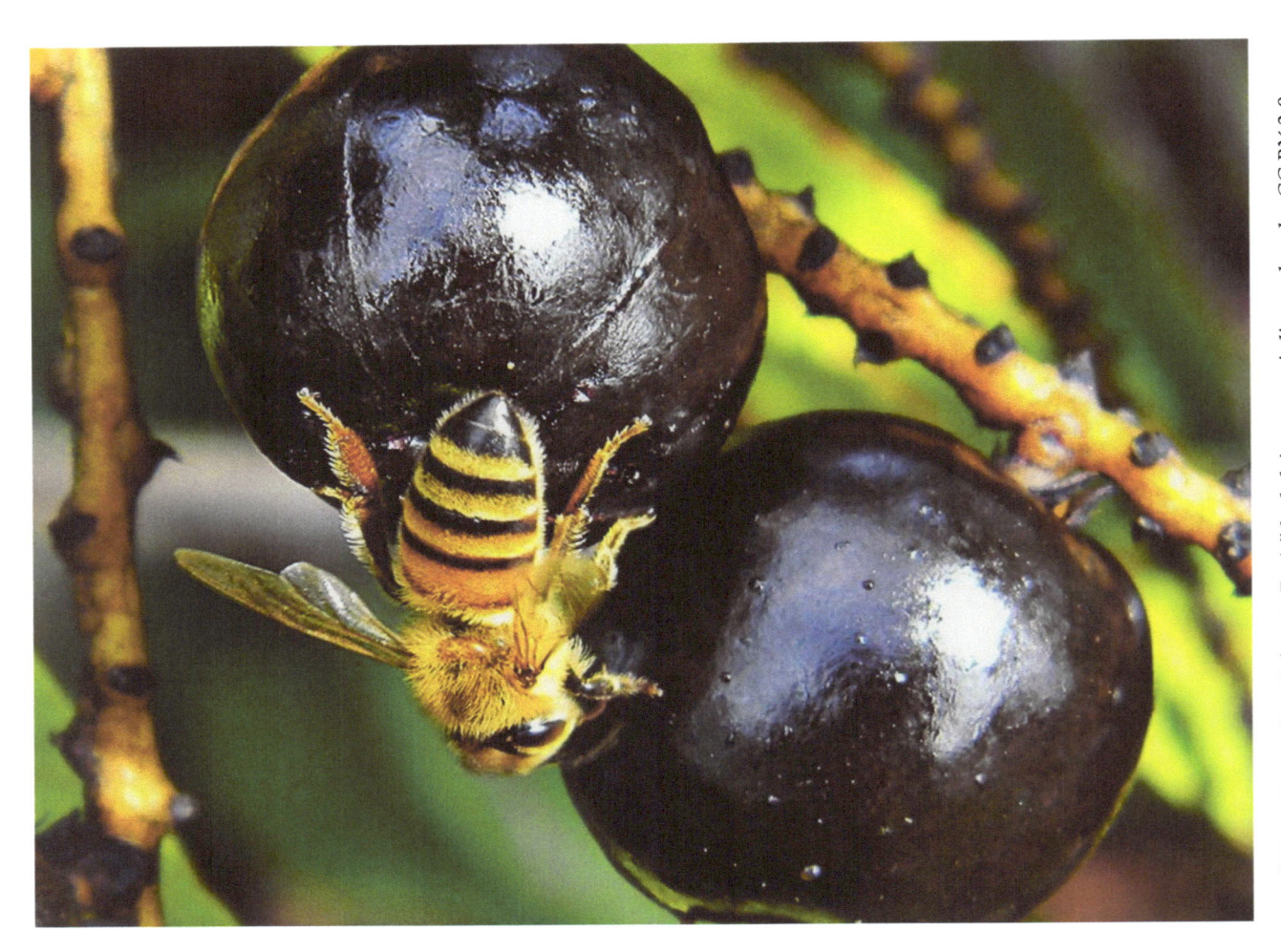

*"Honey Bee on Saw Palmetto Fruit" by bob in swamp is licensed under CC BY 2.0*

Saw palmetto is a small palm tree found in Florida and parts of other southeastern states. It has long, green, pointed leaves like palm trees and branches with small berries.

Native Americans from the Seminole tribe in Florida traditionally ate saw palmetto berries for food and to treat urinary and reproductive problems associated with an enlarged prostate gland. They also used it to treat cough, indigestion, sleeping problems, and infertility.

Saw palmetto treats:

Low sperm count
Low sex drive
Hair loss
Bronchitis
Diabetes
Inflammation
Migraine
Prostate cancer

Sources:
- Androgenetic alopecia. (2015, August) ghr.nlm.nih.gov/condition/androgenetic-alopecia
- Prager, N., Bickett, K., French, N., & Marcovici, G. (2002, April). A randomized, double-blind, placebo-controlled trial to determine the effectiveness of botanically derived inhibitors of 5-alpha-reductase in the treatment of androgenetic alopecia. *Journal of Alternative and Complementary Medicine, 8*(2), 143-52
- Saw palmetto. (2016, June 21) nccih.nih.gov/health/palmetto/ataglance.htm
- Treating female pattern hair loss. (2015, December 9). Retrieved from health.harvard.edu/staying-healthy/treating-female-pattern-hair-loss
- Arca, E., Açıkgöz, G., Yeniay, Y., & Çal??kan, E. (2014). The evaluation of efficacy and safety of topical saw palmetto and trichogen veg complex for the treatment of androgenetic alopecia in men. *Turkish Journal of Dermatology, 8*(4), 210. doi:10.4274/tdd.2302 researchgate.net/publication/272396329_The_Evaluation_of_Efficacy_and_Safety_of_Topical_Saw_Palmetto_and_Trichogen_Veg_Complex_for_the_Treatment_of_Androgenetic_Alopecia_in_Men

# *Mulberries*

## (Morus alba L.)

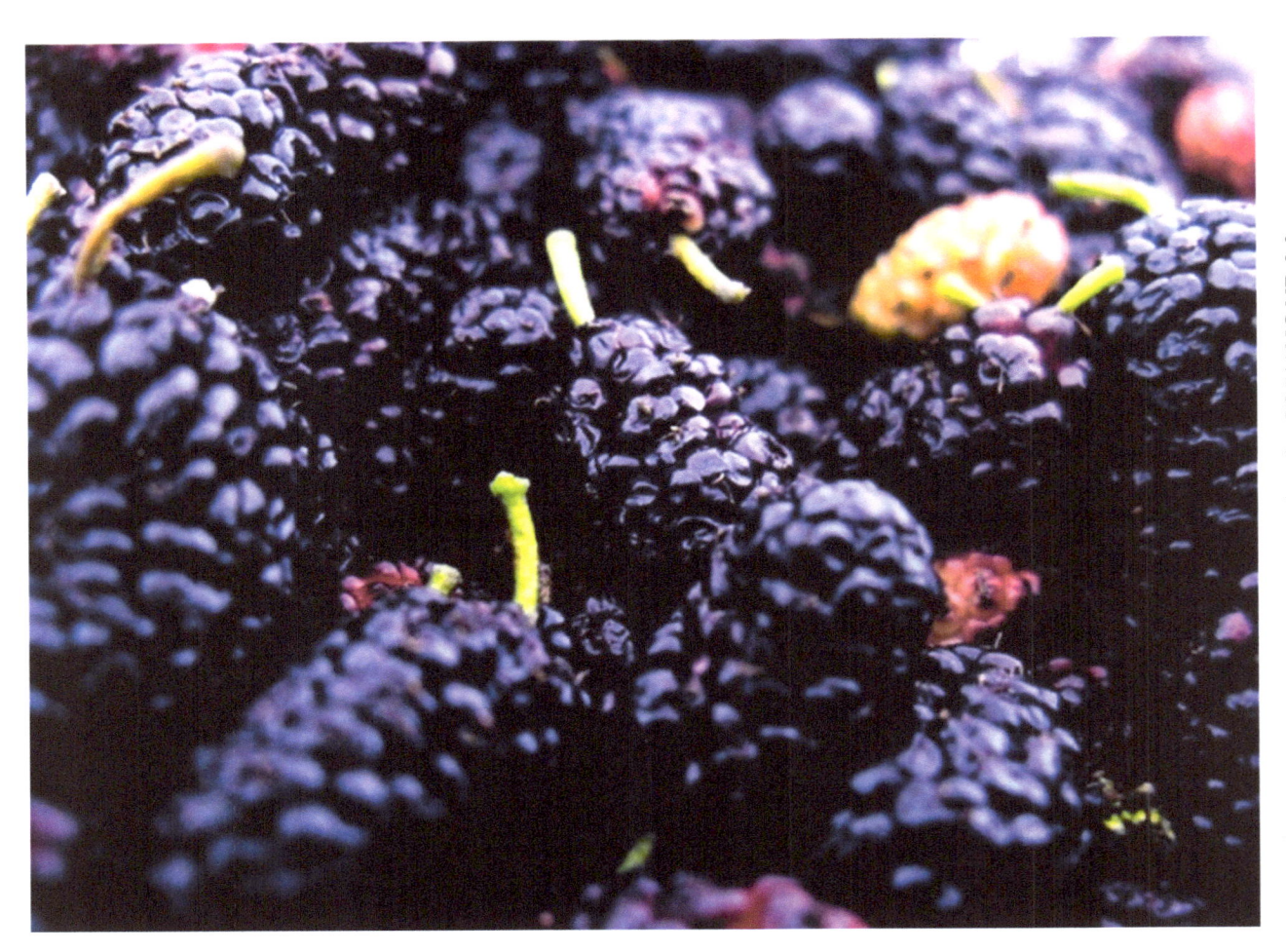

Photo: "Mulberry" by Jean Big Cat licensed under CC BY-NC-ND 2.0

A delicious berry historically used in traditional medicine and ancient healing practices in Africa, Asia, Europe, India, and the Americas.

Improves eyesight
Protects against liver damage
Traditional treatment for diabetes
Anti-tumur
Rich in alkaloid and flavonoids
Powerful antioxidant
Rich in anthocyanins
Protective against cardiometabolic risks as a potent:

Antihyperglycemic
Antihyperlipidemic
Antiobesity
Antihypertensive
Antioxidative
Anti-inflammatory
Anti-atherosclerotic
Cardioprotective

**Sources:**

- Thai Pitakwong, T., Numhom, S., & Aramwit, P. (2018). Mulberry leaves and their potential effects against cardiometabolic risks: a review of chemical compositions, biological properties, and clinical efficacy. *Pharmaceutical biology*, *56*(1), 109–118. https://doi.org/10.1080/13880209.2018.1424210
- Zhang, H., Ma, Z. F., Luo, X., & Li, X. (2018). Effects of Mulberry Fruit (*Morus alba* L.) Consumption on Health Outcomes: A Mini-Review. *Antioxidants (Basel, Switzerland)*, *7*(5), 69. https://doi.org/10.3390/antiox7050069

# Blueberries

## (Vaccinium corymbosum)

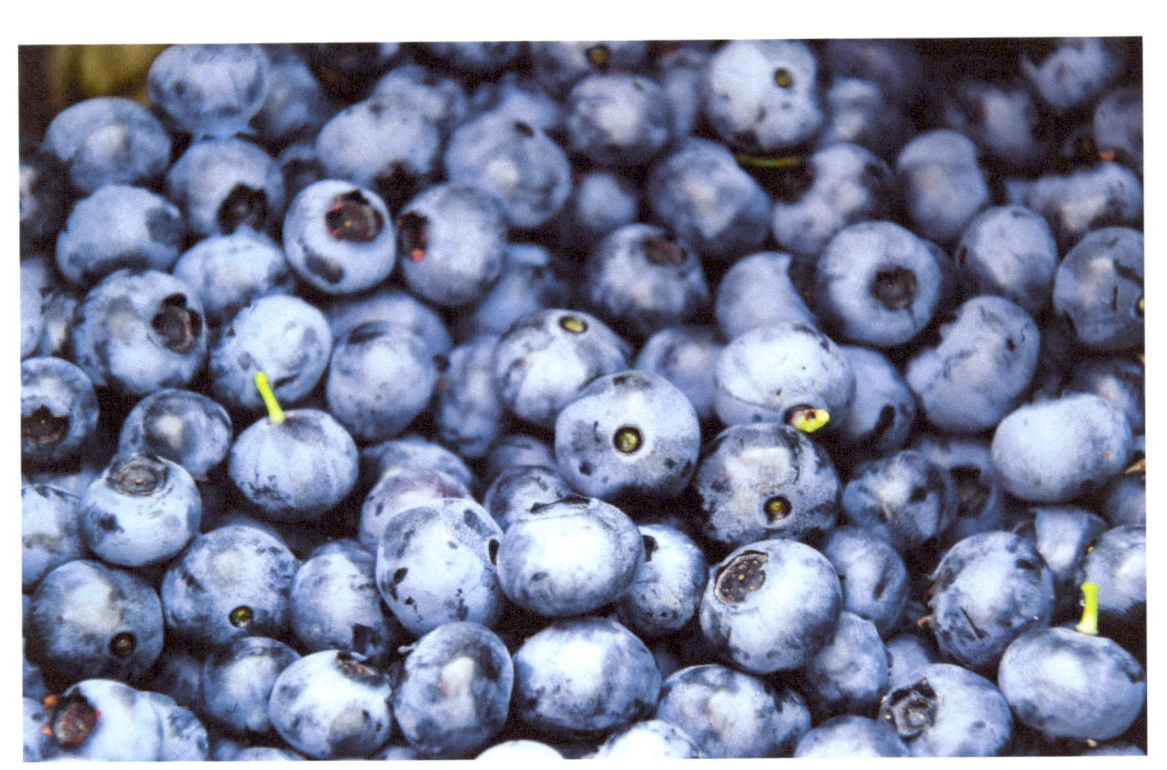

*Photo: "Reward for work: Blueberries" by @rsseattle licensed under CC BY-SA 2.0*

Blueberries contain large amounts of nutrients such as fiber, potassium, and Vitamins K and C. There are many science-backed benefits of blueberries, including boosting antioxidant levels, reducing cholesterol, and improving insulin activity.

Health Benefits:

Low in calories and high in nutrients
The king of antioxidant foods
Reduces DNA damage, which may help protect against aging and cancer
Protects cholesterol in your blood from becoming damaged
Lowers blood pressure
Helps prevent heart disease
Helps maintain brain function and improve memory
Anthocyanins in blueberries may have anti-diabetes effects
Helps fight urinary tract infections
Reduces muscle damage after strenuous exercise

Source:

Wilhelmina Kalt, Aedin Cassidy, Luke R Howard, Robert Krikorian, April J Stull, Francois Tremblay, Raul Zamora-Ros, Recent Research on the Health Benefits of Blueberries and Their Anthocyanins, *Advances in Nutrition*, Volume 11, Issue 2, March 2020, Pages 224–236, https://doi.org/10.1093/advances/nmz065.

# Blackberries

## (Rubus fruticosus)

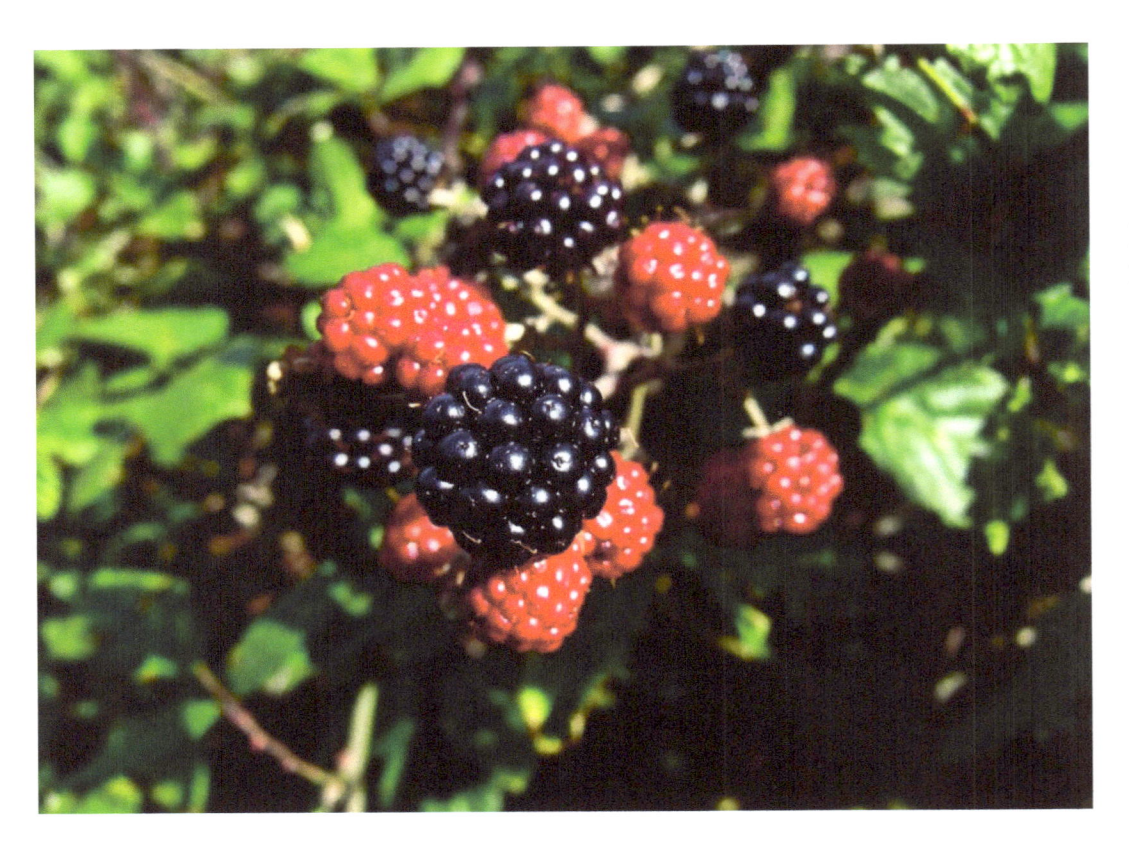

*"Blackberry" by Lastaii licensed under CC BY-NC-SA 2.0*

Rich in protective plant compounds called anthocyanins, vitamins, and minerals, these deep purple berries are packed with goodness.

Health Benefits:

High in fiber
Packed with Vitamin C
Excellent source of Vitamin K
High in manganese
Boosts brainpower and health
Supports oral health
Protective against heart disease
Anti-inflammatory

Source:

https://www.bbcgoodfood.com/howto/guide/health-benefits-blackberries

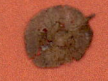

## Section IV:

## Liberation Entrees, Main Courses, and Meals

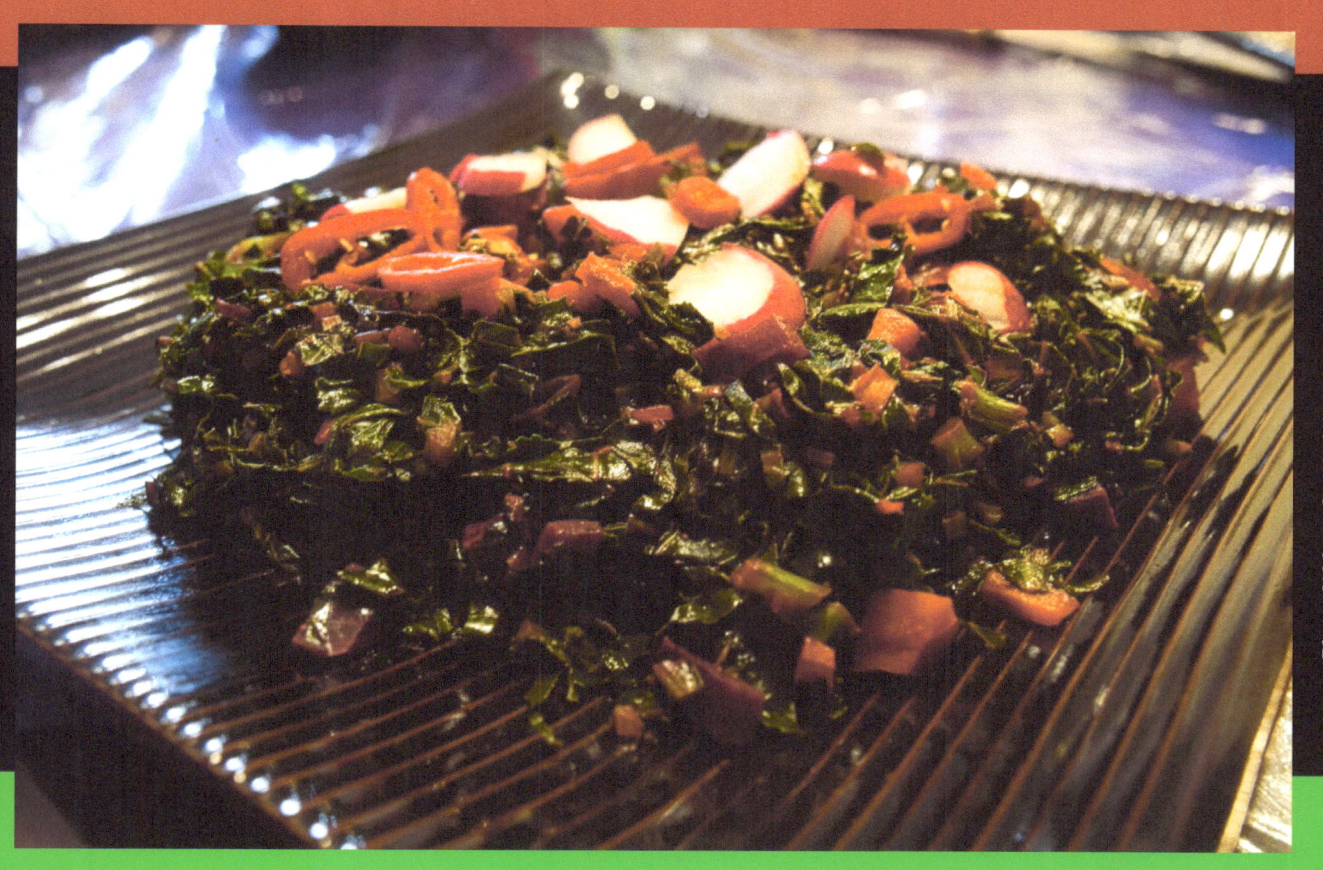

*Photo: Wekesa O. Madzimoyo*

# Black-Eye Peas Quick Liberation Lunch

## Mama Afiya

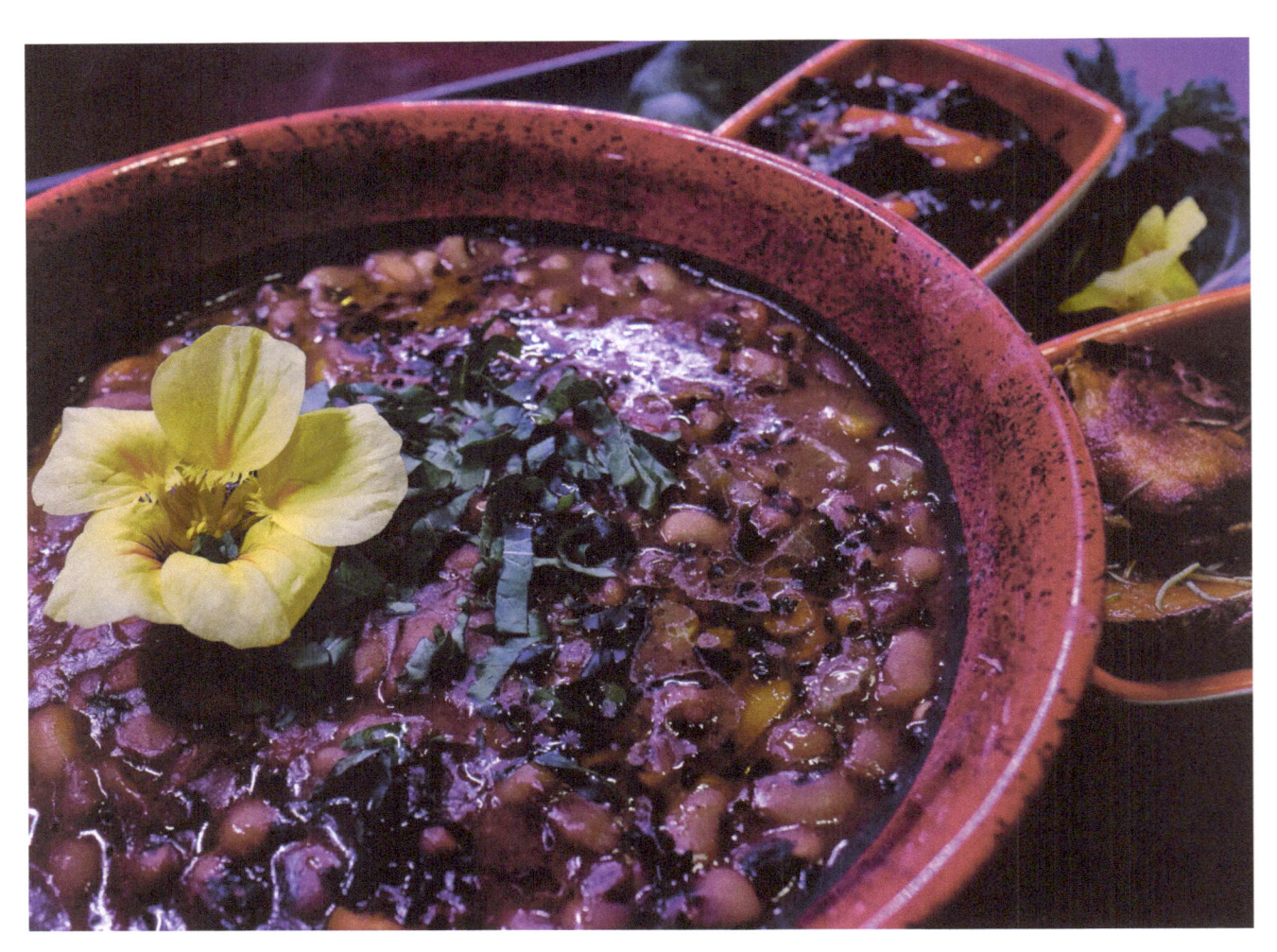

*Photo: Wekesa O. Madzimoyo*

Nicely seasoned black-eye-peas garnished with chopped arugula and nasturtium; Malabar spinach and sweet potato leaf with red pepper; pan-seared sweet potato with rosemary

## Ingredients for Black-eye Peas

- 2 cups black-eye peas cooked and still firm (cooked ahead or in Instapot for 15-17 minutes) left in pot liquor
- 2 tablespoons coconut Oil
- Sweet red, yellow, and green peppers (one of each)

- 2 stalks celery
- 1 large carrot
- 1 clove fresh white garlic
- ½ small onion
- Large green onion scallion
- 1 inch-sized fresh ginger
- ¼ teaspoon salt
- 1 teaspoon country barley miso
- ½ teaspoon fresh or dried sage
- ½ teaspoon fresh or dried thyme
- ½ teaspoon ground cumin

## Directions:

Place coconut oil into a pot. When the oil is hot, place chopped peppers, celery, carrot, garlic, onions, and ginger in, and then let simmer. Saute chopped veggies until crisp and tender. Add in cooked peas, pot liquor, and barley miso. Bring to a boil and reduce heat to a simmer. Add herbs and continue simmering to your desired consistency and taste.

## Ingredients for pan-seared sweet potatoes

- 2-3 medium-sized sweet potatoes sliced 1/4" thick
- 1-2 tablespoons extra virgin olive oil
- Fresh or dried rosemary leaves

## Directions:

In a frying pan, put enough olive oil to pan-fry the sweet potatoes. Place the rosemary leaves on top of the potatoes. Turn. Prevent the rosemary from burning. Finish with the rosemary side up with the bottom side slightly blackened. Be careful, as olive oil burns quickly.

## Ingredients for Malabar Spinach and Sweet Potato Leaf Stir-Fry

- 3 cups Malabar spinach roughly chopped
- 1 cup sweet potato leaves roughly chopped
- ¼ tsp sea salt
- 1 small onion roughly chopped
- 1 tablespoon finely chopped garlic
- 1 small red bell pepper roughly chopped
- Coconut or peanut oil

## Directions:

In wok or skillet, place your oil which can take the most heat without burning. Avoid olive oil. Turn the heat as high as it will go. Before the oil is at a burning point, add in spinach, sweet potato leaves, and other veggies. Stir fry the leafy greens until they are slightly crunchy. Salt to your taste.

# Blueprint for Black Love Dinner

## Mama Jasmine

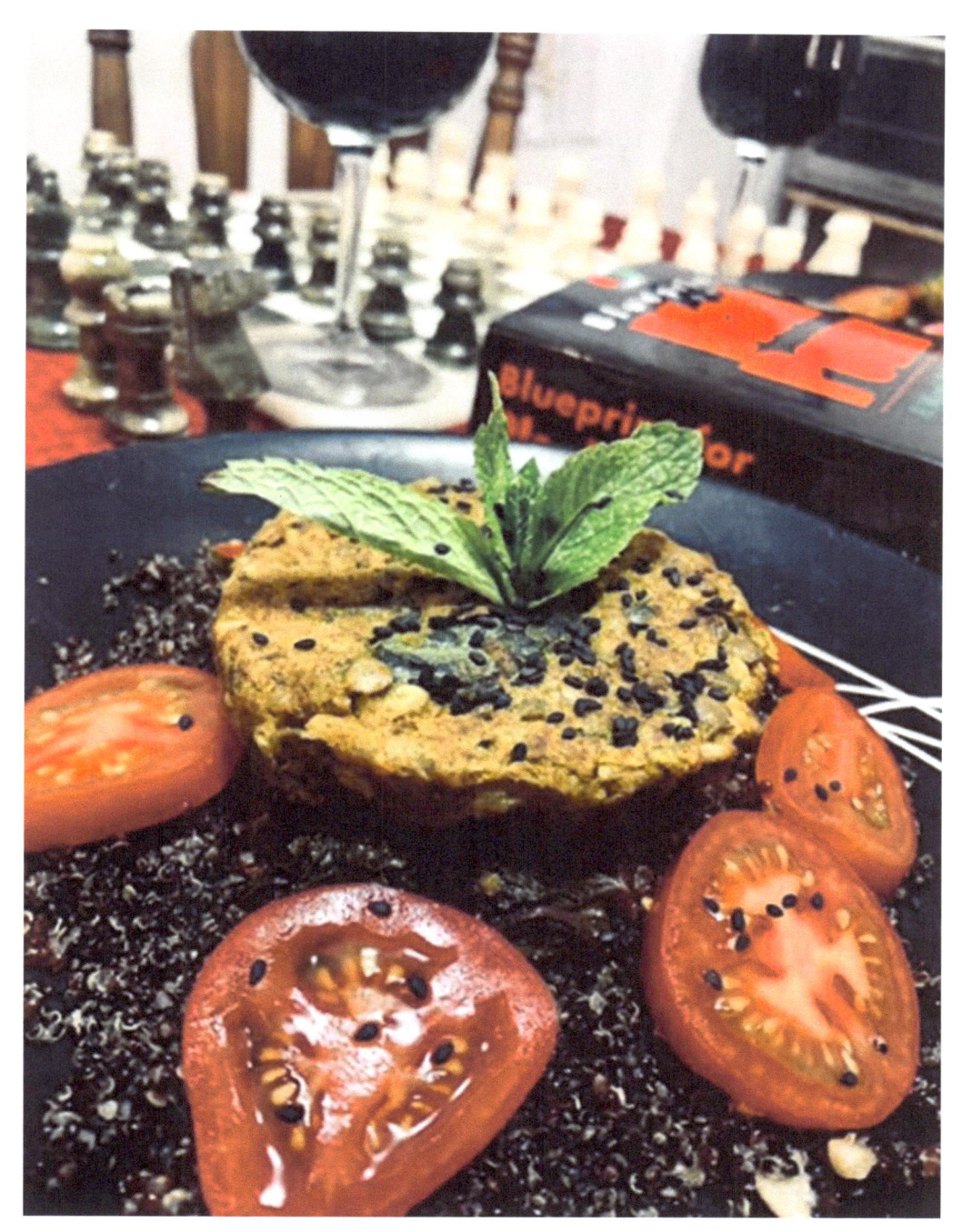

*Photo: Jasmine Barber*

## Ingredients:

- Madras Curry veggie burger by No Bull Burger (https://nobullburger.com/)
- Organic red quinoa
- Organic black quinoa
- Fresh or frozen spinach
- 2 tablespoons freeze-dried garlic (can also use fresh garlic cloves)
- ¾ cup chopped purple onions
- Bragg's Organic Sprinkle 24 Herbs and Spices
- 1 tablespoon Grapeseed oil
- Fresh tomatoes
- Organic mint
- Sesame seeds
- Blk Water, for beverage (https://shop.getblk.com/)

## Preparation:

Prepare black and red quinoa according to package directions.

Add ¼ cup of chopped onions and 1 tablespoon of fresh garlic or freeze-dried garlic slices to the boiling water for extra flavor.

While quinoa is simmering, heat the lentil curry patties according to package directions.

Pan saute spinach with garlic, onions, Grapeseed oil, and season with Bragg's Organic Sprinkle.

## Plating:

Place spinach in a small mound in the center of the plate. Toss the quinoa with grapeseed oil. Surround the spinach with black and red quinoa. Place the lentil curry pattie on top. Place freshly sliced Roma tomatoes along the side. Sprinkle black sesame seeds and top with mint as a garnish. Serve with a glass of Blk Water and Lots of Black Love!

# Black Rice with Roasted Vegetables

## Mama Jasmine

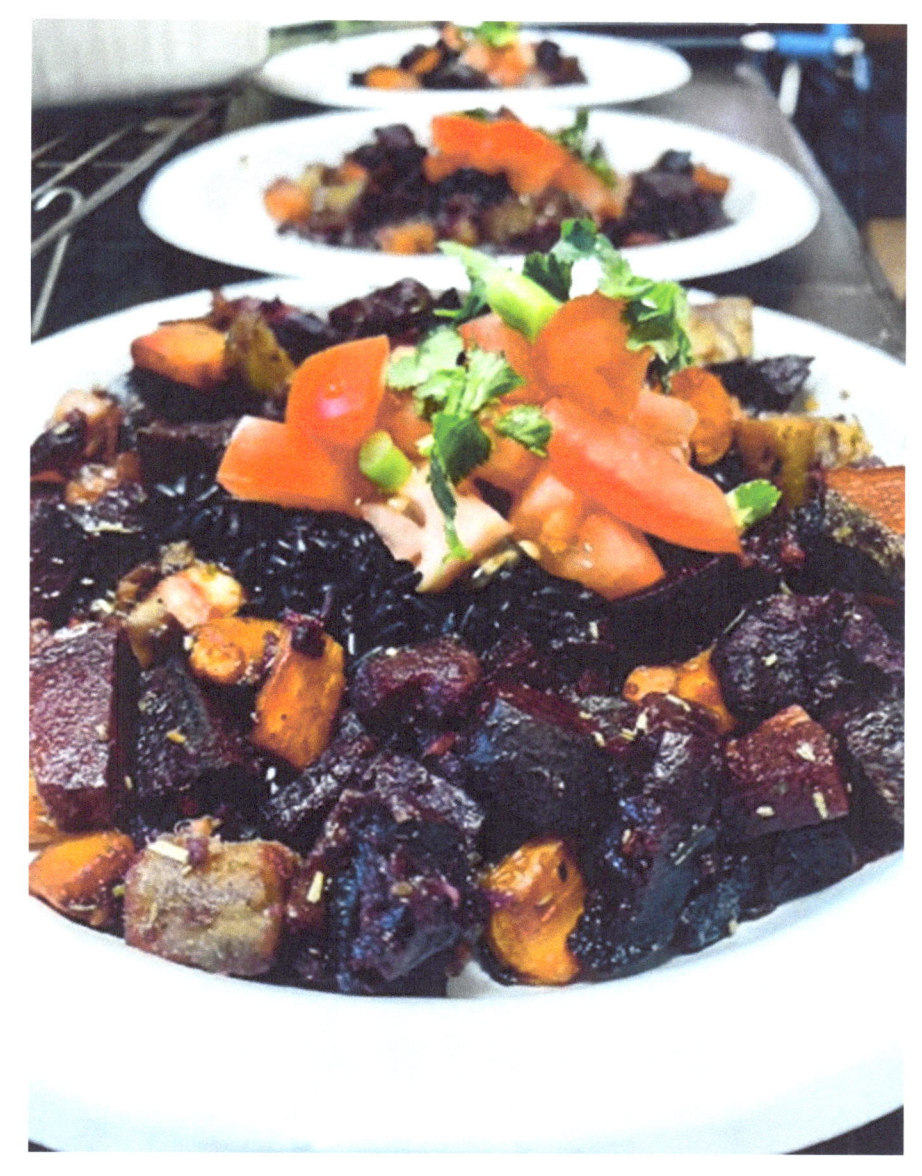

*Photo: Jasmine Barber*

## Ingredients:

- 2 cups black rice cooked (recommended: Lotus Foods Organic Forbidden Black Rice)
- 3 purple sweet potatoes cubed with skin on
- 2 beets, cubed
- 1 whole daikon radish, cubed

- Avocado oil
- Bragg's Organic Sprinkle 24 Herbs and Spices
- Cilantro (for topping)
- 2 tomatoes, chopped (for topping)

## Preparation:

Preheat oven to 400 degrees F. Prepare black rice according to package instructions.

Place cubed root vegetables into a baking dish; season with Bragg's Organic Sprinkle, and drizzle with avocado oil.

Roast root vegetables for 45 minutes to 1 hour until done.

## Plating:

Place a heaping serving of black rice on the center of the plate. Encircle the black rice mound with the roasted vegetables. On top of the mound, place chopped tomatoes and cilantro.

# Grandma Muh's Southern Smothered Collard Greens

## Mama Afiya

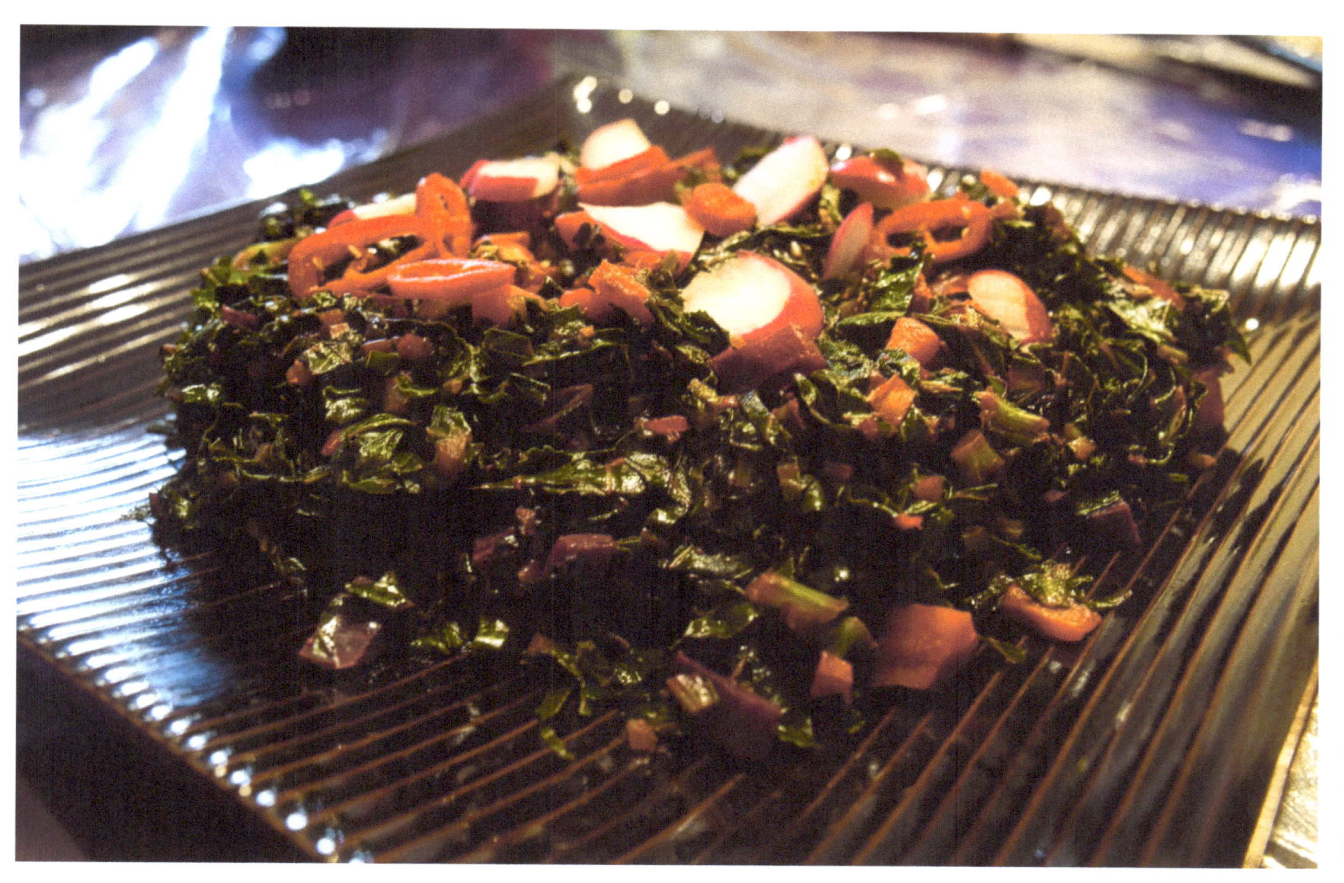

*Photo: Wekesa O. Madzimoyo*

*My Mom made us a leafy green vegetable practically every day. She cooked collards, cabbage, kale, mustard, and rape as part of our "balanced" meals. Folks have always marveled at how the busy, working mother could do this without washing and cooking the greens for hours. She used my Grandma Muh's washing, ribboning and smothering method.*

## Ingredients:

- A mess o' collards
- 1 small green pepper
- 1 small red pepper
- Hot pepper to taste (I like jalapeno)
- Small celery stalk

- 2 small carrots
- Small garlic clove
- Small onion
- 1 tablespoon ginger grated or to taste
- 1 tablespoon chopped sundried tomatoes
- Plant-based oil of choice (I use olive or coconut)
- Chickpea miso
- ¼ cup water
- Coconut aminos
- Pinch of baking soda
- Chopped sweet red pepper
- Chopped red radish

## Directions:

First, clean a mess o' collards by running each leaf under running water. Set aside.

Chop finely green pepper, red pepper, leaving seeds inside. Chop some hot pepper (jalapeno or your favorite to your taste). I sometimes use celery, carrots, and anything else to enhance the color, flavor, or crunch. Essential if you can: chopped fresh garlic, onions, and grate some ginger to your taste. Sun-dried tomatoes are good too. Chop all your veggies finely.

Place collard leaves on top of one another and roll up lengthwise. Cut very thinly, and you will wind up with ribbons.

Saute the other finely chopped veggies on medium-high heat in about 1/4 cup of plant-based oil (I use olive or coconut) to cover the bottom of your pot.

Once the sauteed veggies become soft and a little bit brown, fold in the collards and increase your heat to almost high. The water from the collards will create good steam.

Take 1 tablespoon miso and mix it into ¼ cup water. Stir until dissolved. Place it into the pot and mix it in nicely.

Sprinkle in about five shots of coconut aminos. Add salt to your taste. Let greens cook for 10 - 12 minutes; place a tiny pinch of baking soda in, and shut off the heat. The greens will continue cooking and softening deliciously. Garnish with sweet red pepper rings and chopped red radish.

# Roasted Cauliflower Steak with Poblano Peppers

## Mama Afiya

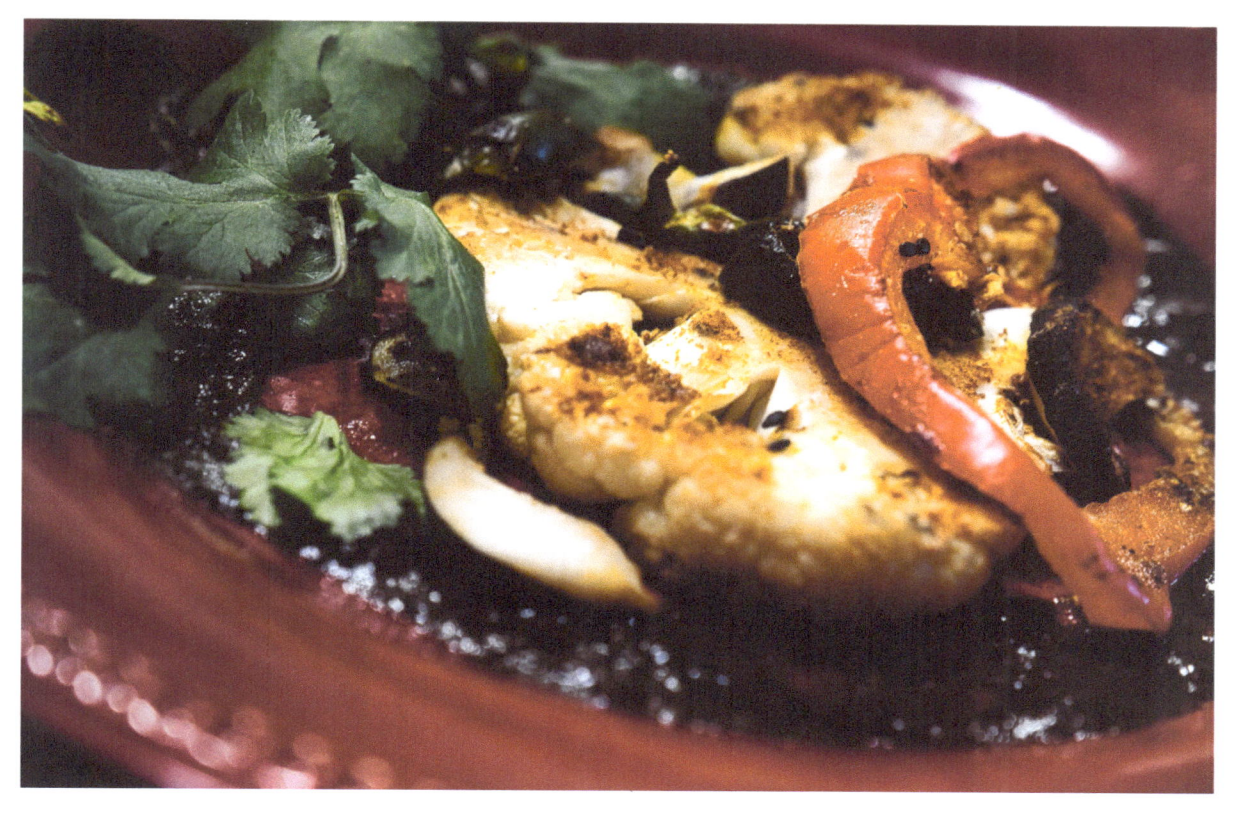

*Photo: Wekesa O. Madzimoyo*

## Ingredients for Roasted Cauliflower

- 1 head cauliflower
- 1 thinly sliced zucchini
- 1 thickly sliced poblano pepper
- A few jalapeno peppers (to taste if desired)
- A few black radishes roughly chopped
- Black sesame seeds
- 1 teaspoon cumin powder
- 1 teaspoon curry powder
- ½ cup nutritional yeast
- ⅛ cup olive oil

## Ingredients for Black Garlic Gravy

- 1 small sweet onion
- 3 green onion scallions
- 1 Garlic clove
- 1 Clove black garlic (for a twist, try ½ teaspoon black garlic powder)
- ¼ cup coconut oil
- ¼ cup brown rice flour
- 1 tablespoon chickpea miso whisked in 1 cup water
- 1 splash San J Soy Sauce
- ½ teaspoon Cuban (or regular) oregano (fresh or dried)
- Sea salt to taste

## Directions:

Roast the cauliflower:
Slightly coat the roasting dish with olive oil, and then assemble cauliflower and other veggies and seasonings onto it. Drizzle a little olive oil on top of the veggies. Bake at 425 degrees for up to 20 minutes, ensuring not to overcook the cauliflower. Broil quickly to give cauliflower a good browning.

Now, let's make the gravy.
Chop both onions and both kinds of garlic finely. Saute in a saucepan in coconut oil. When chopped veggies are translucent, stir in brown rice flour and saute. Add miso water, a splash of soy sauce, and sea salt to your taste. Add oregano; simmer on very low for a few more minutes.

To assemble, place the roasted cauliflower and other veggies onto a plate; place the gravy around the perimeter; garnish with fresh cilantro.

# Artichoke Pizza with Love

## Mama Habiba

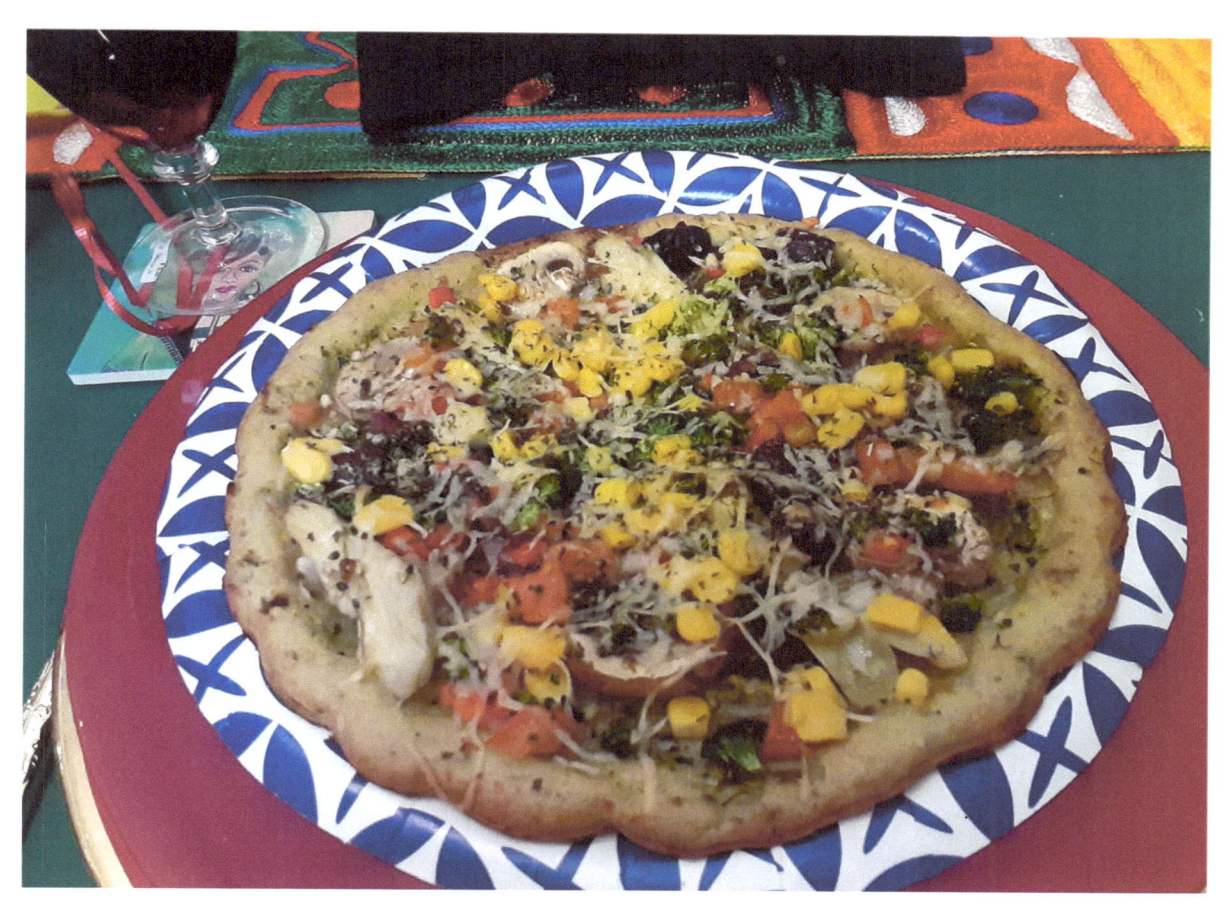

*Photo: Habiba Hall-Bey*

**RED** bell pepper and onions, tomatoes
**BLACK** olives, mushrooms
**GREEN** broccoli, jalapenos
with artichokes, corn, garlic, cheese and a lot of Love
Cauliflower crust

# Sassy Vegan Pizza

## Mama Cheptu

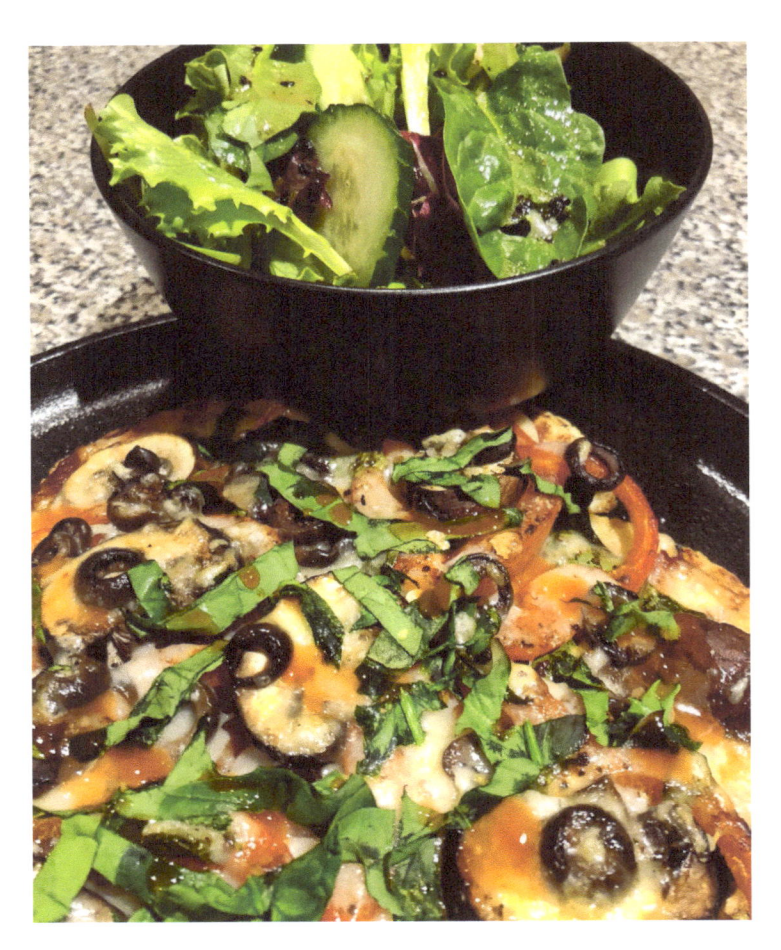

*Photo: Grace Cheptu*

**RED** bell pepper, tomato paste, and see that sassy hot pepper sauce on top?
**BLACK** olives, baby portobello mushrooms
**GREEN** spinach, basil, herbs
Vegan mozzarella holds everything together
Cauliflower/almond flour crust

# Black Love Day Dinner
# Pan-Seared Salmon with Black Bean Pasta and Salad

## Mama Cheptu

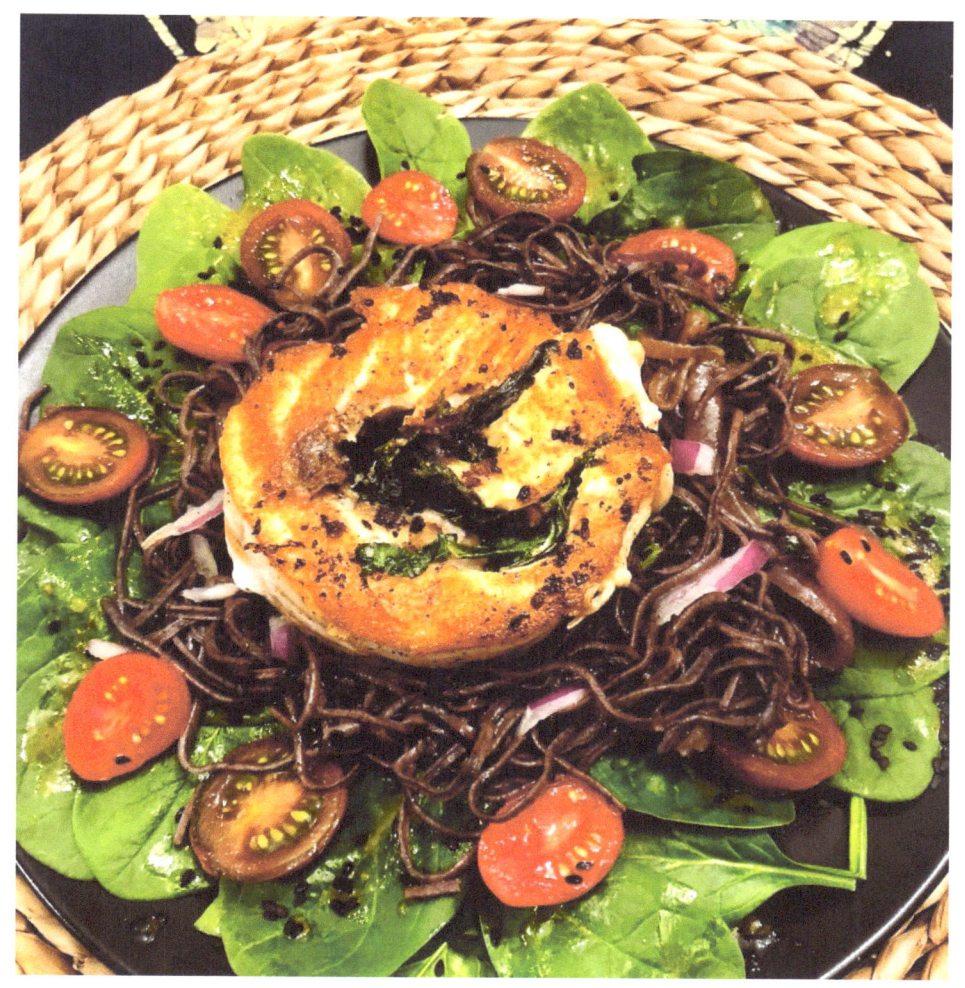

*Photo: Grace Cheptu*

## Ingredients for Pan-Seared Salmon:

- 1 (2.0-pound) center-cut boneless, skinless salmon fillet
- 1½ cups vegan cream cheese* (see alternative recipe below)
- ½ teaspoon fine sea salt divided into half
- 1 tablespoon Dijon mustard
- 1 cup packed baby spinach divided into half

- 2 teaspoons chopped fresh dill
- 2 teaspoons chopped fresh oregano
- ½ teaspoon ground black pepper divided into half
- Lemon juice for sprinkling
- Extra-virgin olive oil for searing

## Directions:

Butterfly salmon fillet through the center, without cutting all the way through, so that it lays open flat in one large piece like a book. Turn salmon over so that the skin side is facing up and place on a clean work surface.

Season salmon with ¼ teaspoon of the salt and ¼ teaspoon of the pepper, dill, and oregano, then spread fillet with mustard. Arrange half of the spinach on top, leaving a 1-inch border around the edges. Evenly dot cheese on top of spinach, then top with remaining spinach. Starting from one of the long sides, gently roll up salmon and tie snugly with cooking twine at about 1-inch intervals.

Slice salmon roll into rounds about 1½ inches thick. Secure each round with toothpicks and brush with olive oil. Sprinkle both sides with the remaining salt, pepper, dill, and oregano. Discard twine that falls off.

Heat pan to medium-high and add oil. Sear salmon "steaks" for about 2 minutes on each side. Allow resting for about 2 minutes. Sprinkle with the juice of ½ lemon before serving. Enjoy!

# Homemade Alternative for Store-bought Vegan Cream Cheese:

## Ingredients:

- ⅔ cup cashews soaked in water for at least 1 hour
- ¼ cup water
- ½ teaspoon apple cider vinegar
- ½ teaspoon dijon mustard
- ½ teaspoon garlic powder
- ¼ teaspoon sea salt
- ⅛ teaspoon red pepper flakes

## Directions:

Drain the cashews and add them to a high-speed blender with all the other ingredients. Blend until smooth and creamy.

# Liberation Tian: Eggplant, Tomato, Zucchini

## Mama Cheptu

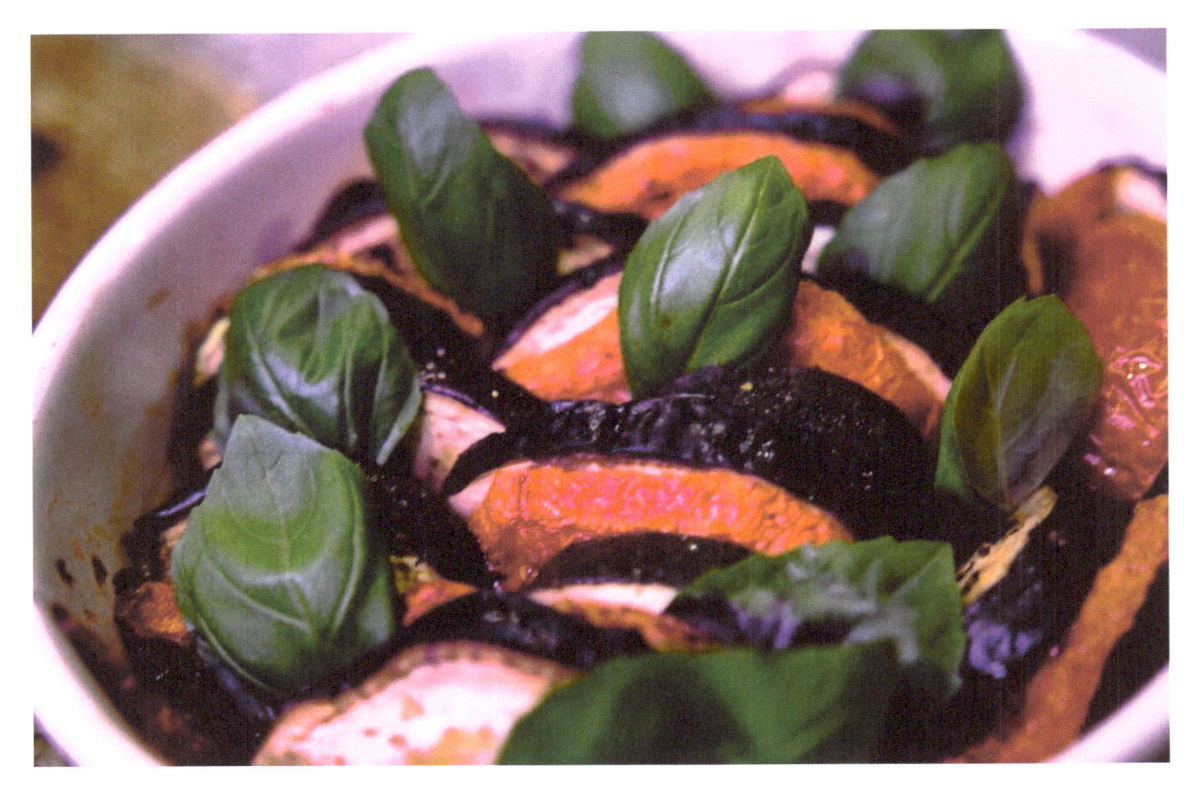

*Photo: Wekesa O. Madzimoyo*

A tian I found online inspired this recipe. A tian consists of vegetables baked in an earthenware dish seasoned with thyme, onions, garlic, and light olive oil. You can use any vegetables you like. I opted for **Red**, **Black,** and **Greens** **for our Liberation Plate Challenge**.

## Ingredients:

- 6 tablespoons extra-virgin olive oil, plus more
- 2 large white or yellow onions, thinly sliced
- Kosher salt and freshly ground black pepper
- 2 teaspoons freshly chopped thyme
- ¼ teaspoon crushed chile flakes
- 6 cloves garlic, minced
- 1 lb. medium zucchini, cut into ¼-inch-thick slices
- 1½ lb. small, firm eggplant, cut into ¼-inch-thick slices
- 1½ lb. ripe tomatoes, cored and cut into ¼-inch-thick slices
- Large leaf "sweet" basil, to garnish

## Directions:

Preheat the oven to 400 degrees F.

Saute onions in oil until translucent. Season with salt and pepper, then add the thyme, chile flakes, and garlic. Cook for 2 minutes more.

Spread the cooked onion mixture onto the bottom of a large earthenware baking dish, about 9 by 13 inches. Arrange the zucchini, eggplant, and tomatoes in alternating rows on top of the onion mixture. Pack the rows tightly so that the vegetable slices stand vertically on their edges. Continue filling the baking dish; then sprinkle with salt and pepper. Drizzle with a little more olive oil.

Bake uncovered for 15 minutes. Reduce heat to 350 F and continue baking for 45 minutes to an hour, or until the vegetables are quite tender. Remove from the oven and let cool to room temperature. Insert a few basil leaves between the vegetable slices to infuse their mesmerizing flavor as the dish cools. When ready to serve, garnish with a few more basil leaves. I like it best at room temperature, and it's even better the next day!

# Steamed Mussels in Garlic and White Wine Sauce

## Mama Cheptu

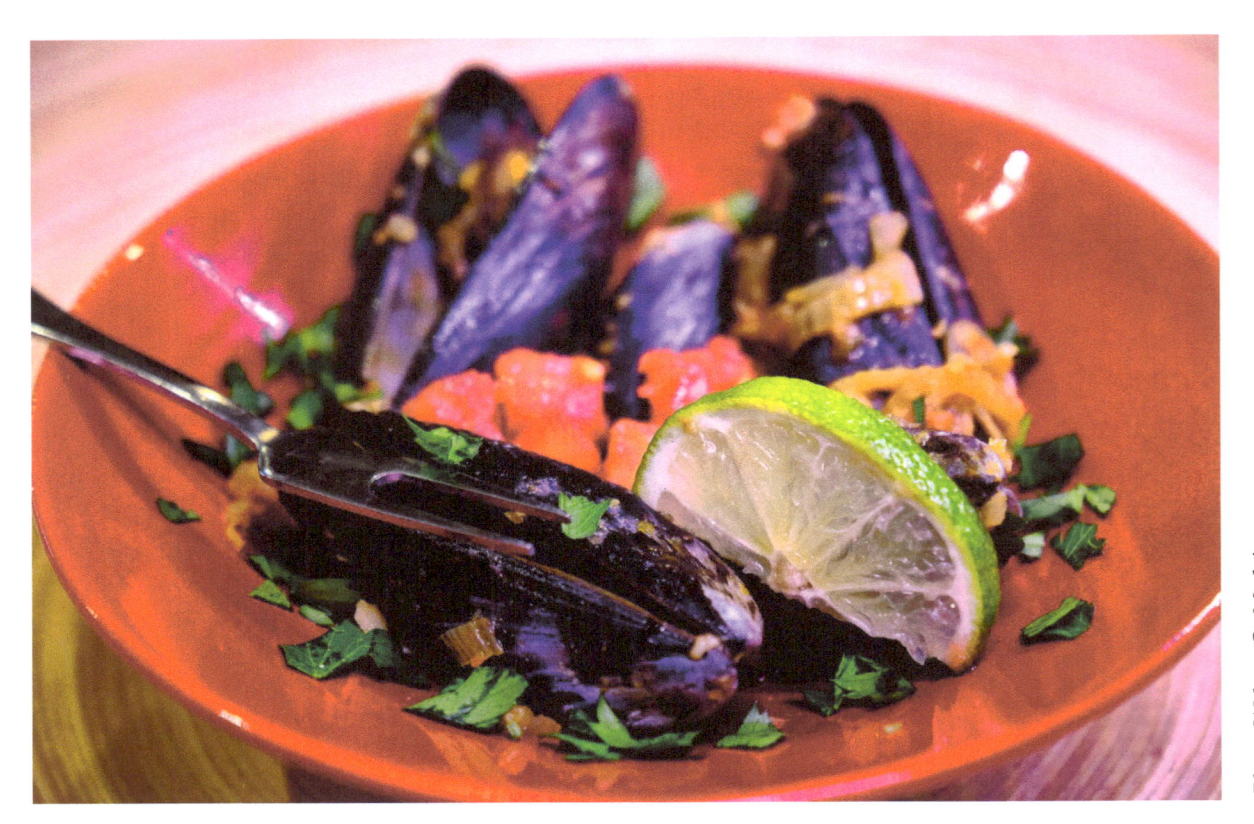

*Photo: Wekesa O. Madzimoyo*

*This recipe traditionally uses lemons and dry white wine. If desired, substitute vegetable broth for the wine. I opted for lime slices to complete our **Red**, **Black,** and **Green** theme.*

## Ingredients:

- 1½ pounds fresh mussels
- 2 tablespoons virgin olive oil
- ½ cup shallots, minced
- 4 garlic cloves, minced
- ¾ cup diced Roma tomatoes
- 1 teaspoon lemon zest
- 2 tablespoons lemon juice
- ½ cup dry white wine (or vegetable broth)
- 4 wedges lime (or lemon)
- Kosher salt and black pepper, to taste
- 2 tablespoons chopped parsley

## Directions:

Scrub mussels under cool running water. Remove "beards," if present, by pulling the fibrous material towards the hinge of the shell.

In a large stockpot, heat olive oil over medium heat. Add shallots and garlic. Cook until translucent/soft, about 2 minutes. (Be careful not to brown the garlic. It will be bitter if browned!)

Add tomatoes, stir and cook, about 2 minutes.

Add wine, lemon zest, and half of the lemon juice, stir to combine.

Quickly add mussels, cover, and steam for 3 minutes. Open and stir.

Re-cover and steam until mussels open, about 2 to 3 minutes.

Taste. If desired, season with the remaining lemon juice, zest, salt, and pepper. Top mussels with parsley and serve with lemon or lime wedges.

If you're a bread eater, toast rustic bread slices to accompany your mussels. You will surely want to dunk them into the succulent broth. Yum-yum!

# Black Pad Thai Noodles and Stir-Fried Vegetables

## Mama Jasmine

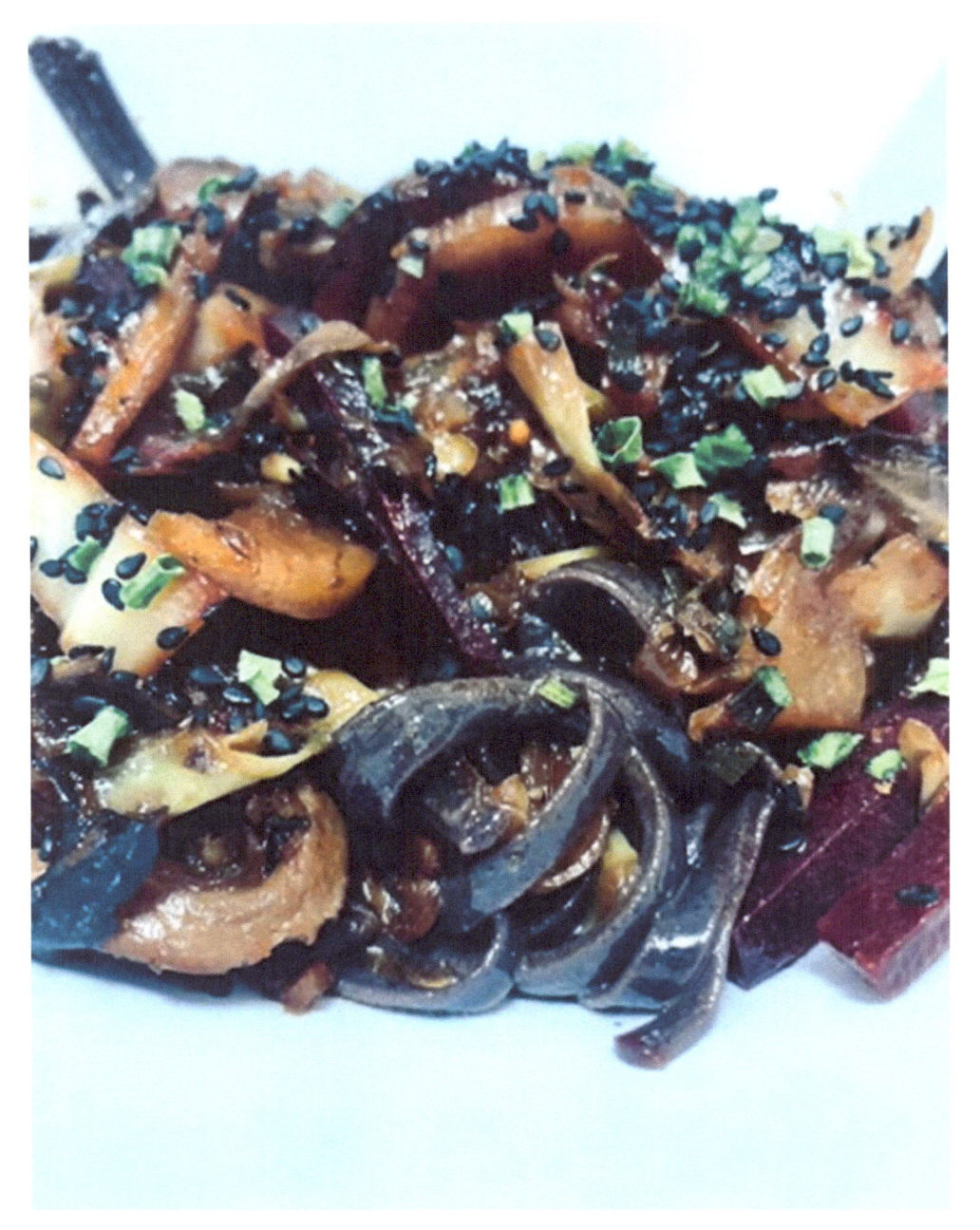

*Photo: Jasmine Barber*

## Ingredients:

- Black pad Thai noodles (Recommended: Lotus Foods Gourmet Organic Forbidden Rice Pad Thai Noodles https://www.lotusfoods.com/)
- 2 beets, sliced
- ½ head of purple cabbage
- 2 cups julienned carrots
- 1 cup sliced shiitake mushrooms
- 1 cup chopped tomatoes
- ½ daikon radish, sliced
- 1 tablespoon Grapeseed oil
- Bragg's Organic Sprinkle 24 Herbs and Spices
- Bragg's Liquid Aminos
- Freeze-dried chives (for topping)
- Black sesame seeds (for topping)

## Preparation:

Prepare black pad Thai noodles according to the directions on the package.

Heat skillet on high heat with Grapeseed oil and saute cabbage, carrots, and daikon radish until tender. Add Bragg's Sprinkle for seasoning.

Add tomatoes, shiitake mushrooms, and Bragg's liquid aminos and heat through.

Add the black Thai noodles to the vegetable mix and add additional grapeseed oil and liquid aminos to the stir fry.

## Plating:

Place the noodle stir fry on your favorite plate. Top with chives and black sesame seeds.

# Grilled Portobello Mushrooms with Avocado Chimichurri

## Mama Cheptu

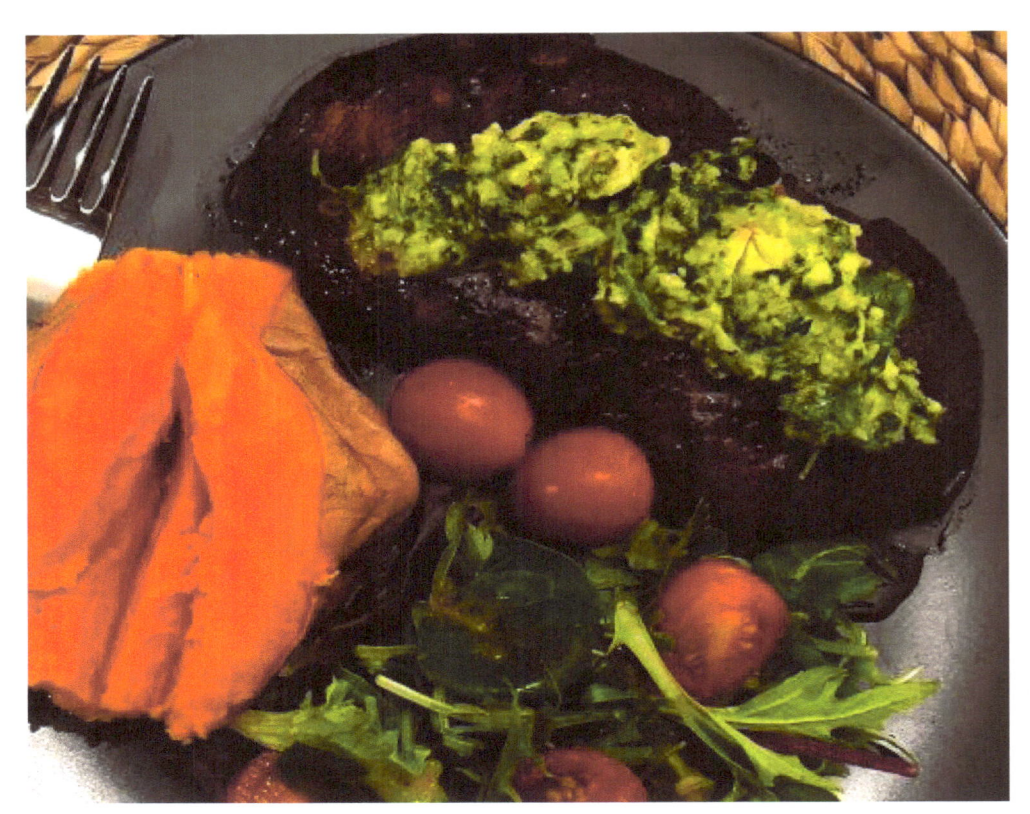

*Photo: Grace Cheptu*

*Several years ago, as I prepared for my traditional Christmas dinner of prime rib with Argentinian chimichurri, my son announced, "I'm vegetarian and won't be eating meat." Oh! Well, okay. Now, I wasn't going to serve him just sides, so I scurried to find something regal that would look and feel like the main entree and feel "beefy" to the palette. Thanks to the "Minimalist Baker," I found a delicious recipe for grilled portobellos with avocado chimichurri. I tweaked my recipe a bit for my southern palette. I rarely eat red meat now, and I've been grilling portobellos ever since!*

## Ingredients for Portobello Mushrooms:

- 3 or 4 large portobello mushrooms
- ⅓ cup balsamic vinegar
- ¼ cup olive oil

- ½ teaspoon cumin
- ½ teaspoon black pepper
- ¼ teaspoon smoked paprika
- 3 cloves garlic, minced
- 1 pinch of smoked salt to taste (sea salt is fine).

## Ingredients for Avocado Chimichurri:

- 1½ cups parsley, finely chopped (flat-leaf is best)
- 3 cloves garlic, minced
- 1 small shallot, minced
- ¼ teaspoon red pepper flakes
- 3-4 tablespoons extra virgin olive oil
- 3 tablespoons red wine vinegar (can substitute lemon juice)
- ½ teaspoon each sea salt and freshly ground black pepper
- 1 small ripe avocado

## Directions:

Remove stems from the mushrooms; then use a spoon to scrape off the "gills" on the undersides. (You can save the stems and gills to flavor broth, soups and stocks.) Wipe mushrooms clean with a dry cloth. Add to a shallow baking dish or plastic freezer bag.

In a small mixing bowl, whisk together vinegar, olive oil, cumin, black pepper, paprika, and salt. Taste and adjust seasonings as needed.

Add sauce to the mushrooms, and be sure that all sides of the mushrooms are covered.

Marinate for 5 minutes, then flip over and marinate the other side for 5 minutes. (Don't exceed 10 minutes, or you'll have soggy 'shrooms!)

Prepare chimichurri by whisking parsley, garlic, shallot, red pepper flakes, olive oil, red wine vinegar, salt, and pepper to a medium mixing bowl. Taste and adjust flavor as needed, adding more vinegar for acidity, salt for flavor, or red pepper flakes for heat.

Add avocado (cut into cubes) and gently toss. Set aside.

Heat grill or cast-iron skillet over medium heat. Cook mushrooms on each side for 2-3 minutes, or until caramelized and deeply golden brown. Brush on any remaining marinade while cooking to infuse more flavor.

Serve with a dollop of the avocado chimichurri.

# Vegan Stir Fry

## Mama Jasmine

*Packed with tender spinach and healthy veggies, this stir fry is delicious. The black rice base gives texture and an exotic flavor. Serve with your favorite kombucha or cup of healing tea for added nutritional benefits.*

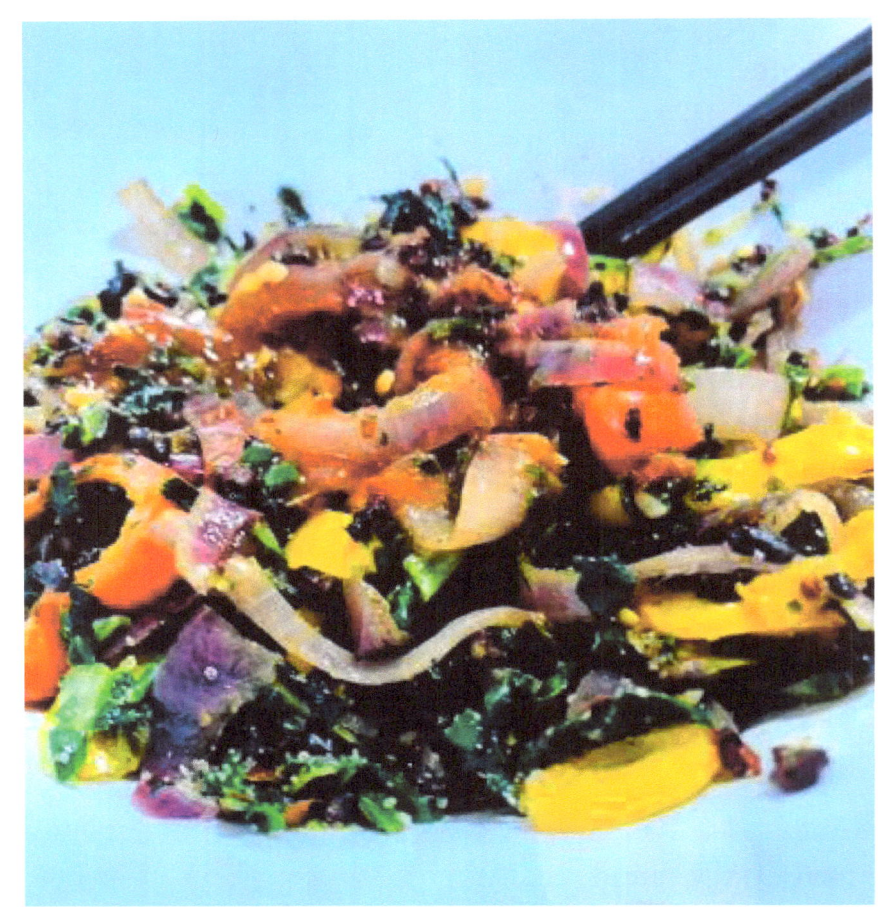

*Photo: Jasmine Barber*

## Ingredients:

- Black rice (recommended: Lotus Foods Organic Forbidden Black Rice)
- 5 spring onions chopped
- 1 red onion chopped
- 1 lb of spinach (fresh or frozen)
- 5 cloves of garlic, chopped
- 2 cups assorted bell peppers sliced
- 1 tablespoon Grapeseed oil

- Bragg's Organic Sprinkle 24 Herbs and Spices
- Bragg's Liquid Aminos
- Red chili paste (optional)
- Red pepper flakes
- Black sesame seeds (for topping)

## Preparation:

Prepare black rice according to package instructions.

While the rice is cooking, heat a skillet on medium-high with Grapeseed oil.

Saute spring onions, red onions, and assorted bell peppers until tender.

Add garlic and spinach and continue to saute with Bragg's Liquid Aminos. Add Bragg's Organic Sprinkle seasoning to taste.

## Plating:

Place hot, steaming black rice into a bowl or onto a plate.

Top with the veggie stir fry.

Add a couple of dollops of red chili paste to your desired level of spiciness.

Sprinkle with red pepper flakes and black sesame seeds.

# Hopi's Yummy Plate

## Mama Hopi

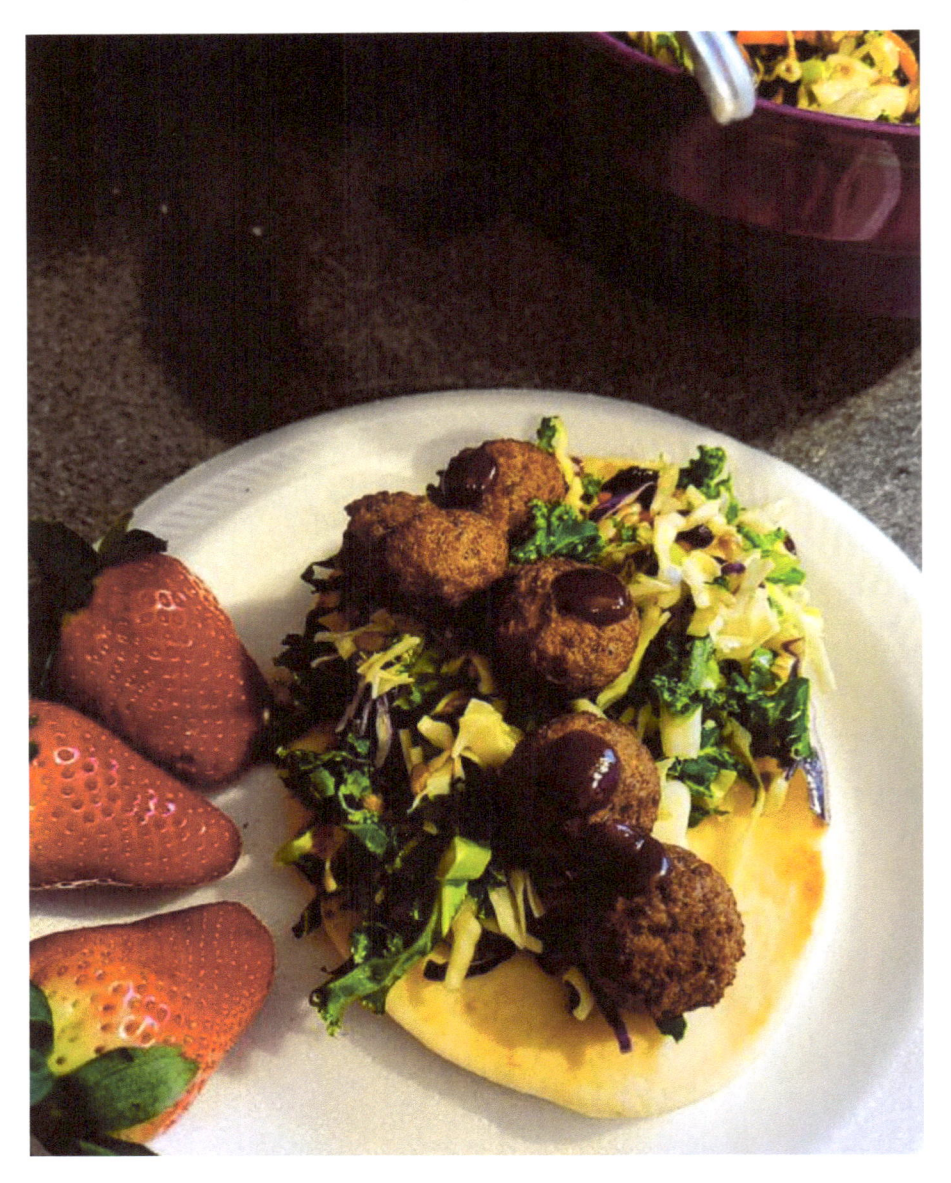

*Photo: Hopi Love*

*I got this delicious recipe from another sister, and it is delicious! You can find all the ingredients at your local grocery store. (I purchased mine from Aldi.)*

## Ingredients:

- Plant-based meatballs (from the frozen section in your grocery store)
- Sweet Kale Crunch Salad Mix (with cranberries, pumpkin seeds, lemon poppyseed dressing)
- Your favorite BBQ sauce
- Naan bread (or pita)
- Strawberries (or any other fruit you like)

## Directions:

Preheat oven and bake meatballs in an oven-safe dish according to package directions for about 25 minutes.

In a bowl, mix all the ingredients for the Sweet Kale Crunch. Set aside.

Lightly toast the Naan in the oven for the last five minutes while the meatballs bake.

To assemble, top the Naan with salad, add meatballs with little dollops of your favorite BBQ sauce. Serve with your side of fruit.

# *Kimchi Black Fried Rice with Black Beans and Organic Pea Leaves*

## Mama Jasmine

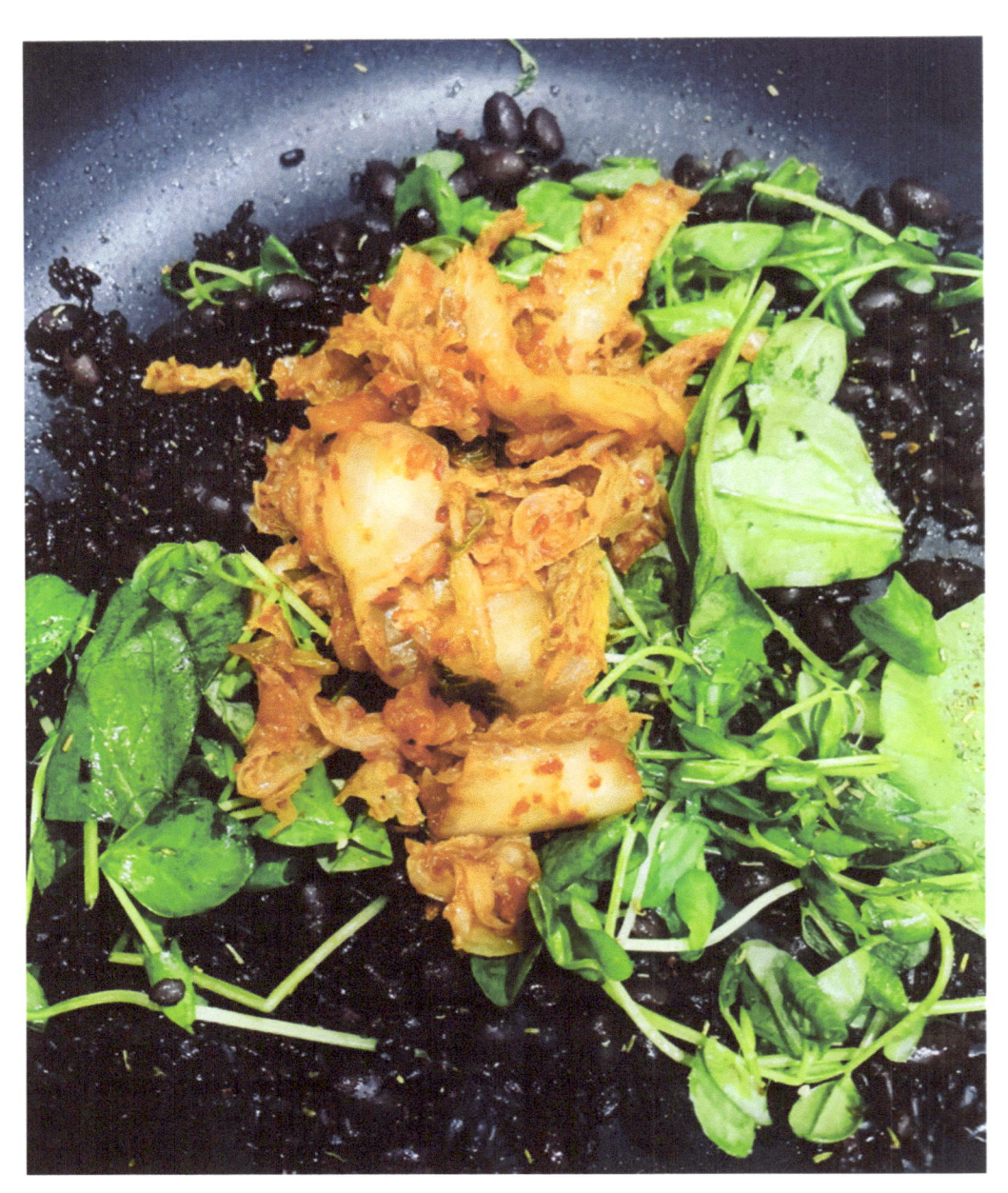

*Photo: Jasmine Barber*

## Ingredients:

- 2-3 cups black rice (recommended: Lotus Foods Organic Forbidden Black Rice https://www.lotusfoods.com/)
- 1 cup of black beans (cooked)
- 1 cup organic pea leaves
- Kimchi (as much as you want for your plate)
- 5 cloves of chopped garlic
- 1 tablespoon Grapeseed oil
- Bragg's Organic Sprinkle 24 Herbs and Spices

## Preparation:

Prepare black rice according to package instructions.

Heat the skillet to medium-high with Grapeseed oil once the rice is done (or use leftover rice).

Place the rice in the skillet and saute.

Add cooked black beans to the skillet and heat thoroughly.

Add chopped garlic and Bragg's Organic Sprinkle and saute for an additional 5-7 minutes.

## Plating:

Place the black rice and bean mixture in a bowl or plate.

Top with organic pea leaves.

On top of the bed of leaves, add as much kimchi as you want.

Sprinkle with black sesame seeds.

# "Barbecued" Tofu with Grilled Asparagus and Black Rice

## Mama Cheptu

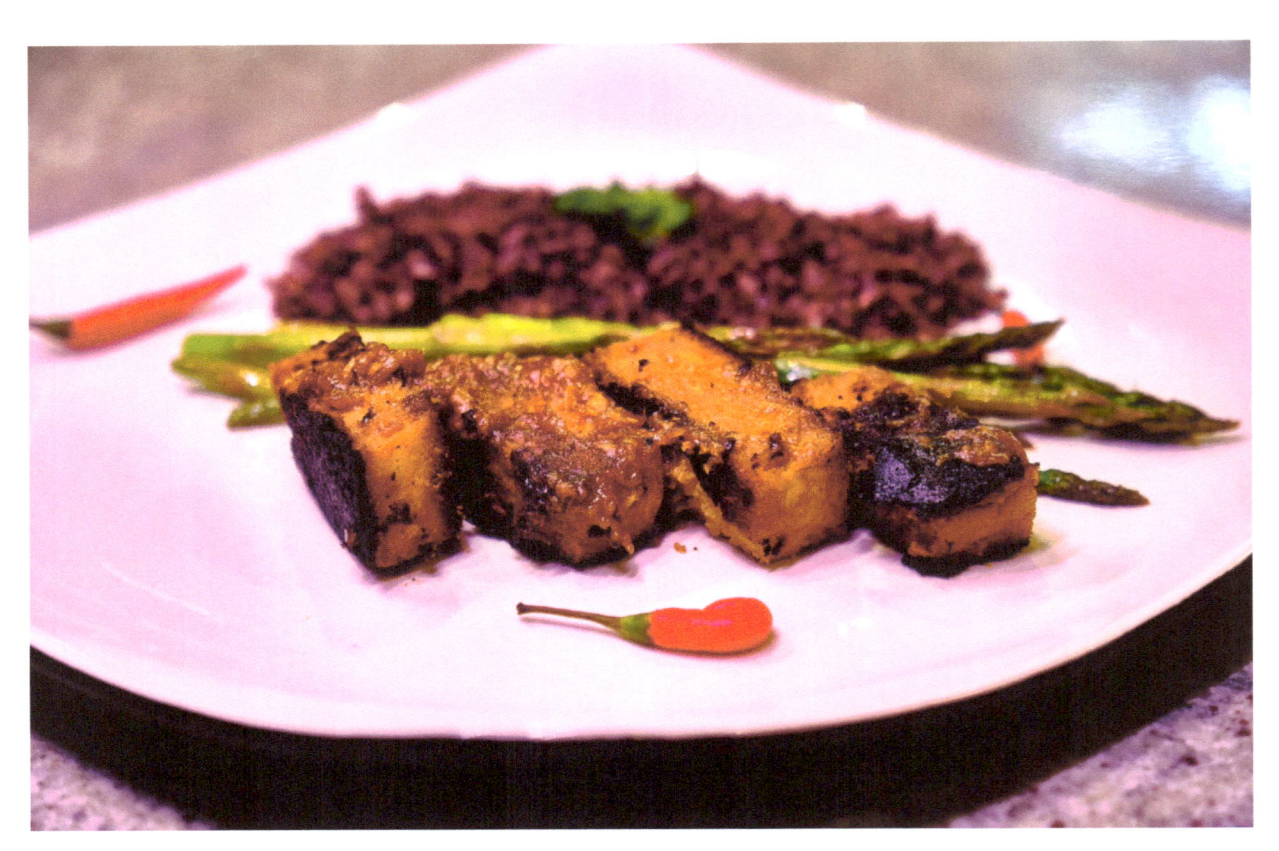

*Photo: Wekesa O. Madzimoyo*

*I love the Thai flavors of this "barbecued" tofu: the ginger, garlic, tamari, and crunchy peanut butter make for a tasty and spicy bite. And the tasty charred "barbecued" bits will leave you wanting more! A tip for hearty textured tofu that can soak up a lot of favor: Freeze your block of tofu when you bring it home from the store. Thaw in the refrigerator overnight when ready to use it, then press out the water. To press out the water, start by wrapping the thawed tofu block in a clean dish towel. Set it onto a plate with something heavy on top like a cutting board or another plate - not too heavy because you don't want to squash the tofu. Press 20 minutes to an hour. Or you can do it the way I did it: just carefully press the water out with the palm of your hands. In 2-3 minutes, I was done! This tofu will now be ready to soak up the flavors of all your delicious ingredients.*

## Ingredients:

- 10 oz. extra firm tofu
- 3 tablespoons organic maple syrup
- ¼ cup tamari sauce
- 1 tablespoon freshly squeezed lime juice
- 3 tablespoons sesame oil, divided
- 1-2 tablespoons Sriracha sauce (depending on how much heat you like)
- 3 tablespoons natural crunchy peanut butter (you can substitute other nut butters)
- 2 garlic cloves (minced, microplaned, or grated)
- 2 teaspoons of fresh ginger (grated or microplaned)
- Lime wedges, toasted peanuts, basil, or cilantro for garnish

## Directions:

Preheat the oven to 350 degrees F. Cut the tofu into 1" cubes and place on a parchment-lined sheet pan. Bake for 20 minutes to dry out the tofu.

Meanwhile, whisk the maple syrup, tamari, sesame oil, lime juice, sriracha sauce, peanut butter, garlic, and ginger in a small bowl. Stir in the baked tofu and marinate for 10-30 minutes.

Warm a medium non-stick saute pan on medium heat with 1 tablespoon of sesame oil. Using a slotted spoon, transfer the tofu to the pan. Some of the marinade will transfer to the pan, which is desirable. Cook tofu on medium heat, allowing it to get a little crispy with some crust forming from the marinade. Gently turn to form a crust on all surfaces. (Saute a total of 5-8 minutes, depending on how "crispy" you like your crust). Set aside and keep warm. You can warm some of the leftover marinade to slather over the tofu just before serving. The leftover marinade can be frozen and used again.